DISCOVER ANDROGRAPHIS

Alex Panossian, Ph.D., Dr. Sci.
with
Terry Lemerond

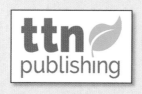

Copyright © 2020 TTN Publishing, LLC, Green Bay, WI

Library of Congress Cataloging-in-Publication Data is on file with the Library of Congress.

ISBN: 978-1-952507-02-1

Design: Gary A. Rosenberg • www.thebookcouple.com
Editor: Kathleen Barnes • www.takechargebooks.com

Printed in the United States of America

10   9   8   7   6   5   4   3   2   1

Contents

PART 1

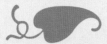

Your Immune System, Andrographis and its Allies

CHAPTER 1

A Primer on
Your Immune System

All of us know what it's like when we get run down. Maybe your life has been more stressful than usual. Maybe your diet has lately been less than ideal. Maybe your exercise regimen has fallen to the wayside. All of those elements of everyday life add up to physiological stress, meaning your body is getting overwhelmed. Of course, this can also be psychologically stressful, adding to the load on your body as well as your mind.

When you get run down, for any reason, your immune system may not function as well as it should.

You know the feeling. Maybe you've got a scratchy throat and the sniffles. Or you're just exhausted and it's hard to get out of bed in the mornings. Maybe it's something worse and you're spiking a fever, coughing and showing symptoms of a very serious viral infection.

While infection, especially viral infection, is hard to avoid once it becomes widespread, there is a great deal you can do to prevent weakening your immune system, as well as revving up the infection-fighting engines if you do get sick.

What is the immune system?

This is a very basic primer.

Your immune system is a complex network of cells, molecules, tissues and organs that monitor your body and team up to respond to anything they perceive as an attacker. It defends against infection by a broad range of microbes: bacteria, viruses, fungi and other pathogens called antigens. If the invaders get past the first line of defense, which recognize and destroy them by components of the innate immune system, the immune system finds, destroys and categorizes them. If these antigens try to invade again, components of the adaptive immune system, including the antibody barrier, will keep them out for the long term.

A group of specialized white blood cells with tongue-twisting "cyte" names includes leukocytes, phagocytes and lymphocytes. These and their offspring are the first and last lines of defense against infection-causing invaders, recognizing when you are under attack and remembering former enemies and blocking them before they can attack you again.

Each one works in a different way like a well-harmonized "orchestra" to identify enemy pathogens, track them, wipe them out and stop them from returning. B-lymphocytes generate antigen specific proteins, so-called antibodies, that recognize an attacker and prevent it from gaining a toehold a second time. That is called "adaptive immunity." This is also how vaccines work, giving the immune system just enough of an antigen attacker to trigger an adaptive immune response (antibodies) without actually making you sick.

Types of immunity

Let's back up for a moment and look at the various types of immunity. All of us have three types of immunity:

🐾 **INNATE IMMUNITY:** This is the immune system we are born with. It includes natural barriers (like your skin) and an inborne ability to determine when you are under attack. When the innate immune system runs amok and thinks non-threatening substances like pollen are threatening, it can cause immune system overreaction, resulting in allergies and even serious autoimmune diseases.

❧ **ADAPTIVE OR ACQUIRED IMMUNITY:** This is the immunity you develop throughout your life when you're exposed to diseases, like the chicken pox you had as a kid, that protects you from getting chicken pox again for your entire life.

❧ **PASSIVE IMMUNITY:** Temporary immunity from other sources, like the natural resistance infants get from breast milk or the immunity that comes from vaccines.

Your immune system cells and molecules are found throughout your body, especially in the bone marrow, thymus gland, spleen and lymphatic system.

But here's something that will blow your mind: A large number of those infection-fighting leukocytes reside in your gut or digestive system. Your gut also houses the vast majority of your body's immune response to digested food. Stay with us for a moment here: The conversation between your immune system and the 30 trillion microbes that live in your body starts at birth, in your gut. If your immune system and your gut microbes have a healthy relationship, your immune system is nurtured and you have a healthy immune response. If not, you may have low resistance to all kinds of infections.

WHAT YOU NEED TO KNOW

➤ Your immune system resides in several parts of your body including your gut or digestive system, spleen, thymus gland, lymphatic system and bone marrow.

➤ It is your barrier against all types of infection–causing microbes: bacteria, viruses, fungi and more.

➤ Immune system cells and molecules recognize foreign substances and decide whether you need to be protected from them. They have several lines of defense, starting for keeping you from being infected at all to help fight off an infection once you're sick to protecting you from being attacked by the same pathogens in the future.

CHAPTER 2

Andrographis:
The King of Bitters

I f we told you there is an herb, used effectively for millennia by indigenous people, that prevents and cures anything from the viruses like the common cold and influenza to hangovers to malaria, snakebite, infertility, stomach aches, dementia, heart disease and cancer, what would you think?

You'd probably not believe us. You might think we're crazy or put this book aside. You might even accuse us of selling snake oil, of attempting to sell fraudulent remedies to the gullible.

But what if, in addition to millennia of traditional use, we

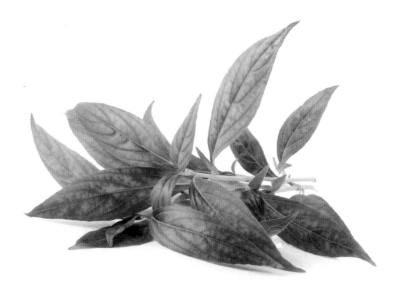

could give you decades of solid modern scientific evidence to prove our claims are true?

That's exactly what we intend to do in this little book. And we believe that by the time you finish reading, you'll wholeheartedly agree that *andrographis paniculata* has a central place in your preventive health routine to strengthen your immune system.

An herb by any other name . . .

Andrographis is central to the herbal traditions of several Asian countries. Today, two-thirds of the populations of developing countries rely on this miracle herb to treat a wide variety of maladies, including viral infections. The herb is known by many names: most commonly as kalmegh, its Bengali name. It's also known as mahatikta or shankini in Sanskrit, kiryato or kariyathu in Gujarati, mahatita in Hindi, nilavembu in Tamil bhooinimo in Urdu, chuan xin lian in Chinese and fah talai jone in Thai. Its multitude of names in so many different languages reflects the importance of andrographis to so many Asian cultures and healing traditions.

In English, andrographis is also often called "The King of Bitters," meaning it tastes extremely bitter, which is why you'd probably want to take it in capsules as it's most commonly found. In herbal traditions around the world, bitter herbs usually have cleansing and temperature regulating effects and improve circulation, benefit the nervous system and cool the body's inflammatory response.

The herb, little known outside of Asia, is also sometimes affectionately called "Andro." Its widespread use in India during the Spanish flu epidemic of 1918–19 is credited with stopping the spread of the deadly disease that killed between 50 and 100 million people worldwide.

Andrographis is oftentimes described as a "handsome" hardy

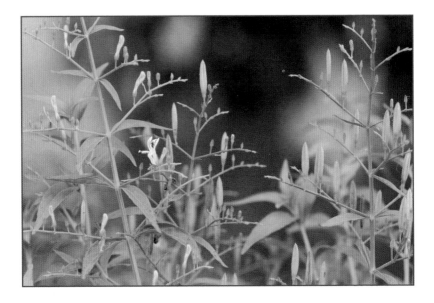

annual shrub, readily adaptable to widely varying soil conditions in its native India and Sri Lanka. Its leafy top reaches as high as three feet with small purple, pink or white flowers. The entire plant, leaves, stem and roots, is medicinally useful. It is often wild-crafted, but Asian organic growers have taken up cultivation in recent years with an eye toward standardized products.

Traditional Uses in TCM and Ayurveda

In Traditional Chinese medicine (TCM), andrographis is classified as a "cold" medicine, helping rid the body of fevers, toxins and heat.

In Ayurvedic medicine, andrographis is similarly considered dry, penetrating and cooling. It is considered kapphapitta, helping remove excess mucous, improving liver function and digestion, and supporting a healthy respiratory tract. Ayurveda is a complex science; so let it suffice to say that these qualities make it one of the most potent of herbs in the Ayurvedic medicine chest. Only curcumin, ashwagandha and holy basil are more widely used in this indigenous Indian medicine tradition.

In both traditions, the primary purpose of andrographis is to support the immune system, but it is used for many, many more purposes because of its ability to maintain homeostasis or biological balance (Yin-Yang in TCM).

Approximately one-third of the world's population lives in Asia where andrographis has been safely used for millennia.

Modern science

Today, andrographis is often associated with fighting colds and flu (and rightly so); it is a "do-everything" herb that may open new pathways toward fighting various infectious diseases (e.g. Lyme disease and malaria), cancer, heart disease, arthritis, other inflammatory diseases, and more. We'll go into this more in Section 2.

As is often the case, the effectiveness of medicines that have been used and revered by indigenous people for millennia is now affirmed by modern science. By the mid-2020, the National Library of Medicine's database returned 971 published studies on the wide spectrum of health effects of andrographis dating as far back as 1951.

Scientific interest in herbal remedies has been high in recent years, specifically in andrographis with 80 studies published in 2019 alone.

Many of the miraculous healing powers of andrographis come from andrographolides, a rare group of diterpenoid lactones, which have strong proven antimicrobial, anti-inflammatory and antioxidant effects. (Andrographis is also a rich source of other nutrients, including well-researched antioxidant flavonoids and polyphenols.)

Andrographolide has been shown to be antiviral against influenza A and avian influenza viruses, herpes simplex virus 1, antibacterial against drug-resistant Staphylococcus aureus, anti-inflammatory for people with rheumatoid arthritis, and anti-tumor against a variety of cancers. Few recent studies suggest direct antiviral effect of andrographolides against SARS coronaviruses. That's quite an impressive list! And that's just to name a few. We'll talk more about that in Chapter 3.

In fact, andrographolide is so well regarded that pharmaceutical companies are even experimenting with synthetic versions of it, a plan that will almost certainly go awry as synthesized versions of natural remedies inevitably do.

With this in mind, our advice is to make sure that the andrographis you add to your regimen delivers natural andrographolide. We recommend a source that includes at least 80 mg (about 1 mg per kg of body weight) andrographolides for a concentrated level of this incredibly versatile compound. More about this later.

Immunomodulation means andrographis regulates the

immune system. It slows down immune function when it's over-active, like we see in allergies and autoimmune diseases. It also enhances immune response when the immune system is unable to stop aggressive infections, leading to viral illnesses including a wide variety of colds and flu. That enhanced immune response also increases Andro's effectiveness against viral and bacterial illnesses and even serious and potentially life-threatening illnesses like cancer, HIV and hepatitis.

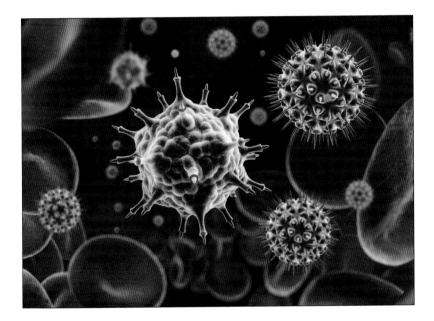

Andrographis is a multi-tasker

That brings us to the concept of adaptogens, the multi-taskers of the plant world. In the simplest possible terms, adaptogens, like andrographis, are plant medicines that provide your body what it needs to increase resistance, resilience and to survive. Adaptogens play a similar role defending your body against environmental challenges, including deadly viruses, harmful bacteria, diseases carried by insects (think of ticks and Lyme disease, mosquitoes and malaria), excessive ultraviolet rays from the sun and challenges from pollution, excess heat and cold, and more.

We think of adaptogens as complex compounds that work as science expands and evolves to better understand the disease process. Adaptogens have the potential to provide broad plant-based treatments for complex diseases, chronic conditions and syndromes. This is an amazingly complex series of synergistic interactions of molecular networks and cellular communication systems that quite literally add up to more than the sum of the parts.

Key to understanding adaptogens is the maintenance of homeostasis, the body's internal wisdom that brings all systems into balance, by building resistance to physical, chemical, biological and psychological stressors.

Adaptogens, like andrographis, actually work like stress vaccines to activate the body's defense system and metabolic rate that will reverse the negative effects of stress and restore the body to balance and health.

If your immune system is not functioning properly by overreacting or underreacting to challenges like viral infections, andrographis supports the correct immune response.

On the other hand, if your immune system is overly active, triggering allergies and asthma, or rheumatoid arthritis or lupus, andrographis will lower the immune system response to a normal level.

WHAT YOU NEED TO KNOW

We'll be going into much more detail on the gifts of andrographis in the coming chapters, but here's a snapshot of the conditions that the King of Bitters, with its scientifically validated benefits, works against:

- colds, flu, upper respiratory infections

- virus fighting, including the herpes simplex virus

- infection fighting, including staph, salmonella and MRSA

- malaria and other illnesses caused by parasites

- rheumatoid arthritis and other autoimmune diseases

Best of all, andrographis has been shown to be as effective as prescription drugs and sometimes even more effective, in many animal studies and some clinical studies in humans, all without serious side effects. In combination with some specific other supplements, as you'll see in the coming chapters, the synergistic effects can be truly remarkable. As always, a well-qualified healthcare practitioner can guide you on the best use of andrographis and all-natural remedies for you.

CHAPTER 3

The Virus Slayer

Not only does andrographis bring about balance in the body, it is inarguably your body's most powerful ally against the onslaught of pathogenic challenges launched at it every day.

What does that mean?

That means that andrographis has been proven effective against virtually all types of infections: viral, bacterial, parasitic and fungal.

The antiviral activity of andrographis is due to its ability to stop viruses from reproducing themselves and slowing or stopping the life cycle of bacteria. Andrographis' ability to activate your immune system in several ways can knock out a variety of pathogenic attacks when you are infected.

Conventional medicine will throw a battery of tests at an infection and then tailor the treatment to the type of infection.

The beauty of andrographis is that it throws its power at all types of infections whether they are viral, bacterial, parasitic or fungal. Best of all, you don't even have to know what type of infection you have in order to find healing and you don't risk antibiotic resistance by taking antibiotics for viruses against which they are completely ineffective.

The immune system is a vastly complex network that affects multiple pathways in the body. Any threats to your defenses can result in some extremely difficult-to-treat conditions. Andrographis appears to rise to almost any of these challenges.

Andrographis is probably best known in the West as a botanical that boosts your immune system's ability to defend you against viruses and bacteria.

Indian researchers had discovered that andrographolides can bind to even the most contagious viruses and neutralize them. It's especially interesting to note here that scientists are not usually prone to hyperbole, but this research group dubbed the potential of andro as "awesome."

While we can't say definitively that andro is *the* answer to all of today's viral infections, read on. The body of research confirms its effectiveness against a wide range of other viral infections.

Flu

About 35 million cases of this basket of serious viral infections are diagnosed every year. That means that more than 10% of Americans experience the fevers, body aches, sore throats and cold-like symptoms that accompany the flu. Most people recover from flu in two weeks or less without medical intervention, but for a small percentage, complications like pneumonia can be life threatening. Flu killed about 80,000 Americans in the flu cycle of 2017–18, many of whom already had chronic conditions or were elderly, very young or frail for other reasons.

For the Northern hemisphere, the flu shot is based on scientific projections from the World Health Organization of the coming year's viral strains based on the strains circulating in the Southern Hemisphere.

In the winter of 2019–2020, the flu shots were 45% effective, according to the Centers for Disease Control and Prevention (CDC). Even if you get the flu shot, you still have a 55% chance of getting the flu.

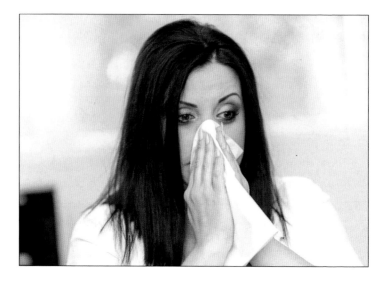

In the terrible flu year of 2018–19, the vaccine provided virtually no protection for the elderly (less than 2%), only about 37% protection for children and adults under 65. Another study, published in 2019, shows contradictory evidence about equal effectiveness of flu vaccine for older and younger flu sufferers.

The vaccine is formulated to prevent several strains of influenza A and B. Each year is different and overall effectiveness rates have been as low as 20% and as high as 67%. Yes, it's a gamble.

So why not improve immune function and prevent colds and flu with andrographis, whether or not you choose to take a flu shot?

A pivotal study from India in 2014 when the H1N1 swine flu was pandemic, showed andrographis had powerful antiviral effects.

Researchers wrote that andrographis has "potent antiviral activity and (as) a potentially new mechanism of action, andrographolide may warrant further evaluation as a possible therapy for influenza."

Here's a brief summary of other research validating andrographis' ability to maximize immune function:

Swedish researchers found that andrographis prevented about twice as many colds than in people who didn't take the herb. Other Swedish research confirms that those who did get colds recovered, especially from sore throat, in about half the time as those who just soldiered on with their colds.

Indian research shows that people who got colds and were treated with andrographis had their symptoms subside within three days, while those who didn't receive the herb were still feeling most of the symptoms at five days.

Andrographis is clearly proven to boost immune function, enabling the body to fight off all kinds of attacks, including viral infections. Indonesian researchers found in 2015 that andrographis stimulated the production of white blood cells called lymphocytes, profoundly increasing the body's abilities to fight infection.

And no wonder: Andrographis helps you get over colds and flu faster and reduces the intensity of symptoms without causing side effects.

You know about the most common viral challenges, the colds and flu that plague most of us every winter. You know the stuffy nose, sneezing and coughing annoyance that usually disappears on its own in a week to ten days, even if you're fairly miserable during the first few days.

In fact, it's estimated that Americans get 1 billion colds a year. That's an average of almost three colds per year for every single American!

About half of all common colds are caused by the rhinovirus, the source of the well-known upper respiratory tract infection—nasal congestion, runny nose, sore throat and cough—that most commonly occurs in the spring and fall. Another 20% or so are caused by one strain or another of the coronavirus, which occurs most often in the coldest months of winter. The remainder, influenza viruses (10–15%) and adenoviruses (5%), can have accompanying gastrointestinal symptoms like vomiting and diarrhea.

In a double-blind, placebo-controlled study, andrographis relieved key cold symptoms in just two days, including fatigue, sore throat, runny nose and sleeplessness. By the fourth day, the andrographis group saw a significant decrease in all symptoms, including headache, earache, phlegm production and coughing.

Another clinical study of individuals with upper respiratory tract infections showed similar results. In this case, 223 patients either received andrographis or a placebo (inert sugar pill). By the third day, there was a dramatic reduction in cough, headache, sore throat and disturbed sleep in those who took andrographis.

Herpes

Now let's get to other viral infections that are far less common, but no less severe and even deadly.

Varieties of the herpes simplex virus cause chicken pox and painful genital herpes, cold sores and shingles. The CDC estimates that as many as 68% of the population has the virus, although it is not active in most people. Herpes simplex is a lifelong virus that stays dormant in the body much of the time and causes periodic eruptions of cold sores, genital lesions and outbreaks of shingles that can last for months or even years.

It's not surprising that the formidable immune protective effects of andrographis suppresses the herpes virus, especially the one that causes cold sores, stopping it from duplicating, according to at least two studies and one in 2011 that suggests andrographis stops the virus from entering cells.

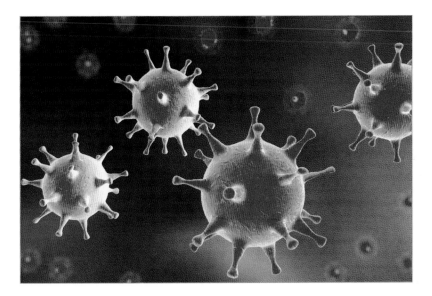

A recent Thai study showed the andrographolides may be more effective at suppressing the herpes virus than conventional pharmaceuticals like acyclovir that can cause blood clots, seizures and more. And Indian researchers found in 2017 that andrographis stimulates several other kinds of cells that selectively target viruses.

HIV/AIDS

Then there's the much-dreaded HIV/AIDS virus. Fortunately, in recent years, science has dramatically reduced the death rate from this devastating disease that destroys the immune system. Human Immunodeficiency Disease (HIV) and Acquired Immunodeficiency Syndrome (AIDS) were a certain death sentence until 1995, 14 years after the disease was discovered.

The CDC estimated in 2015 that 1.1 million Americans age 13 and older were living with HIV, including 152,500 who have not been diagnosed. An estimated 38,500 people are diagnosed with this devastating destroyer of the immune system every year. Since 1987, when HIV/AIDS was first listed as an official cause of death, 507,351 people have died of the disease.

The good news is that the death rate has dramatically declined and many people live fairly long and healthy lives after they are diagnosed with the disease if it is properly treated.

People diagnosed with HIV must take a daily cocktail of antiretroviral drugs for the rest of their lives. The cocktail also reduces the chance the virus will be transmitted through sexual contact or through the birth process.

The drugs do not cure the disease, but the right combination reduces its virulence and stops the virus from multiplying, giving the immune system a chance to recover and be strong enough to fight off infection. There are seven possible classes of drugs that can be included in the cocktail. Most people with the disease take at least two drugs and some must change their drug regimens frequently to stay ahead of the virus' growth.

The reprieve doesn't come without a cost, both material and physical. The drugs are expensive. Some insurance covers much of the cost, other insurance does not. There are some drug assistance programs. Because there are 41 different combinations of drugs that could be included in the cocktail, it is difficult to calculate the average costs of HIV treatment. Some drugs cost as much as $3,000 a month. Some are available as generics, but most are not. The lowest cost of a single drug is $15 a month, but that low cost is the exception, not the rule. The average annual cost of HIV treatment is between $14,000 and $20,000.

The drugs can cause anaphylaxis (severe and life-threatening allergic reactions), liver damage and potentially fatal drug interactions.

Yet, preliminary research suggests that andrographis can be a valuable addition to the drug cocktail and might someday replace some of its ingredients.

Several studies show andrographis increases the body's natural production of infection-fighting white blood cells, to the benefit of HIV/AIDS patients as well as those with any type of infection.

Human research at Washington state's Bastyr University showed that andrographolides significantly increased immune function in HIV-infected people. A Chinese study says andrographis may help boost the function of immune cells and "provides a feasible platform for screening herbal medicine as the treatment for HIV/AIDS."

WHAT YOU NEED TO KNOW

➤ Andrographis has a unique ability to effectively fight all types of infections—viral, bacterial, fungal and parasitic.

➤ Similar effects were shown in prevention and treatment of flu and pneumococcal pneumonia.

➤ The King of Bitters has been clinically proven to prevent the common cold, and in people who were infected with the rhinovirus, it substantially relieved symptoms and reduced the duration of the cold.

➤ Andrographolides have been shown to increase immune function in people with severely compromised immune systems who have HIV and AIDS.

CHAPTER 4

More Power
Against Infections

We mentioned in the last chapter that andrographis has potent powers against all types of pathogens, not only viruses, but also bacteria, fungi and parasites.

Bacterial infections can be really nasty, even life threatening. Ranging from food poisoning to skin infections to venereal diseases, strep throat, urinary tract infections and very serious infections like pneumonia, cellulitis and sepsis, bacterial infections have become more and more difficult to control because of the overuse of antibiotics.

Andrographis is study-proven as an antibacterial warrior, even against bacteria that have mutated as they commonly do when attacked by antibiotics. The most recent Chinese research validates its effectiveness against a wide variety of bacteria and even notes that it can help overcome bacteria that have become antibiotic resistant.

Antibiotics are quickly becoming obsolete because of decades of use, overuse and abuse. Andrographis is becoming a safe and effective alternative.

Andrographis has been confirmed as a potent treatment for bacterial pneumonia (often called pneumococcal pneumonia) caused by the Staphylococcus aureus bacteria. The disease is usually treated with antibiotics or a cocktail of antibiotics and has, in many cases, become antibiotic resistant.

Bacterial pneumonia is a serious disease with a high mortality rate that can spread to the blood, lungs, middle ear or nervous system and demands immediate and appropriate treatment.

Andrographis stops dangerous bacteria like Staphylococcus aureus by preventing it from reproducing.

Andrographolides also enhance the production of infection-fighting white blood cells and helps the lymphatic system eliminate bad bacteria.

Chinese researchers have found that inhaled andrographis, combined with a chemical delivery system called beta-cyclodextrin, could be considered a "potent weapon" against drug-resistant bacterial pneumonia. One study shows it is 91% effective against antibiotic-resistant pneumonias.

Andrographis, a superb immune system enhancer, is even more effective against bacterial infections when it's combined with immune system stimulators, like zinc and vitamin C.

The staph bacteria can also cause skin infections and other serious diseases, including MRSA (antibiotic resistant infection), toxic shock syndrome, impetigo, boils and cellulitis, some of which are fast growing and potentially life-threatening.

Andrographis is being used to treat all of these quickly and effectively.

Lyme Disease

The ability of andrographis to strengthen the immune system makes it an increasingly effective option for treating Lyme disease.

Transmitted by ticks, this bacterial infection by the Borrelia burgdorferi bacteria first manifests itself in "bull's eye" pattern skin lesions, but can later progress to muscle dysfunction, arthritis, facial palsy, stroke-like symptoms and more. It's usually treated with antibiotics.

However, antibiotic treatment doesn't address the need for the body to help heal itself. In fact, Polish researchers found that patients using anti-biotics to successfully treat the skin lesion phase of Lyme disease still had a great deal of free-radical activity, meaning that the bacteria can still cause serious health problems over a long

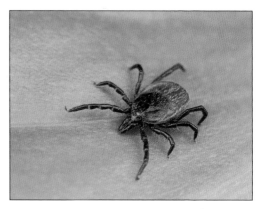

period of time, months or even years.

Antibiotic treatment for these diseases can knock out the acute disease, but there are often long-lasting effects that weaken the system more, creating a greater opportunity for the disease to spread and do more damage. Conventional medicine treats the free radical damage with antibiotics, but antibiotics are ineffective for long-term use.

Over the past several years, the use of andrographis as part of a multi-herbal treatment for Lyme disease, or in conjunction with conventional methods, has grown. There is no reliable research on this subject, but anecdotal evidence suggests it is effective against the post-Lyme symptoms without side effects.

Antifungal

Several studies confirm that andrographis is an effective treatment for fungal skin infection.

Malaysian researchers identified two components of andrographis that are most effective against fungal infections: dichloromethane (DCM) and methanol (MEOH).

Although it hasn't been deeply studied, preliminary research suggests that andrographis could be an effective treatment for Candida albicans yeast infections of the intestinal tract that have a number of causes, including yeast overgrowth from antibiotic use.

Antiparasitic

Malaria affects more than 220 million people worldwide and takes more than half a million lives every year. While malaria is not common in the United States, it is common in tropical and subtropical areas.

Andrographis has been proven to be a powerful weapon against this deadly parasite.

An interesting additional finding from Indian researchers shows that andrographis plus curcumin is even more effective in eliminating the malaria parasite.

WHAT YOU NEED TO KNOW

- ✒ Andrographis can fight all types of infection, including serious antibiotic resistant bacterial infections.

- ✒ Extensive research shows its effectiveness against life-threatening types of bacterial pneumonia.

- ✒ It's also effective against Lyme disease and its complications as well as fungal and parasitic infections.

CHAPTER 5

Melatonin Gives You More Than ZZZs

Here's another part of the immune system equation that may surprise you: Melatonin.

"Melatonin? Isn't that to help you sleep?" you might ask.

Yes, melatonin does help you sleep. A good night's rest is sure to improve immune function as well as overall health. But melatonin's benefits go much farther than simply promoting a good night's rest.

Researchers have long known the link between melatonin and immune function, especially in older people. As we age, our immune systems weaken. That's why common infections like the flu and pneumonia tend to be worse and even more deadly in older people. Aging immune systems sometimes have difficulty differentiating between "bad" pathogens, including bacteria, viruses and more, and the "good" ones.

It's interesting that white blood cells, the first line of defense in the immune system, have melatonin receptors, although scientists aren't exactly sure why. We do know that natural levels of melatonin produced by the pineal gland, the gut and the retina of the eye, diminish as we age. We also know that melatonin helps stimulate the release of cytokines, small proteins that help attack infections and reduce inflammation. We also know that people with the highest blood levels of melatonin are far more able to fight off serious infections.

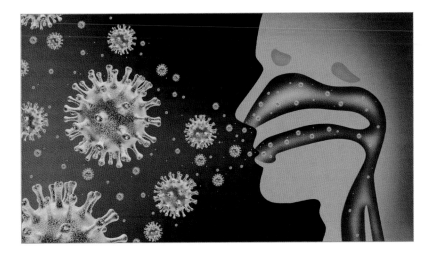

Finally, and perhaps most importantly in today's world, melatonin is a potent antiviral, shown to knock out a wide variety of deadly viral diseases, including SARS, MRSA, avian flu and more. New research strongly suggests melatonin may be a powerful natural weapon against the most serious viruses without serious side effects.

Melatonin's healing powers may be connected to reining in immune system overreaction to viruses and the inflammation that frequently accompanies it, leading to deadly pneumonias and respiratory failure.

As far back as 2005, a multi-national team of researchers concluded that melatonin is a key part of healthy immune function in the elderly and immunocompromised people, those most likely to be infected by viruses.

Andrographis and melatonin

So, what, you might ask, if we put andrographis and melatonin together? You're right on track with a consortium of American scientists who asked the same question and came up with a hopeful answer, as early as August of 2020 in a study published in the journal *Life Sciences*. They concluded, "Considering the properties of both compounds in terms of anti-inflammatory, antioxidant, anti-pyrogenic, antiviral and ER stress modulation and computational approaches revealing andrographolide docks with the SARS-CoV2 binding site, we predict that this combination therapy may have potential utility against (even the most deadly viruses)."

Sorting out the scientific lingo for a moment here, they think the combination of andrographis and melatonin could work together to prevent and treat. As of this writing, we are still early in the pandemic research game, but this is an exciting development that has the potential to save many lives. Stay tuned. We'll update you as more information becomes available.

Read on. There's more, much more.

What exactly is melatonin?

Melatonin has been called a hormone, and indeed it does have hormone-like properties as a chemical messenger. But Dr. Walter Pierpaoli, one of the world's foremost anti-aging researchers, insists melatonin is not a true hormone. He's the first to admit, as a decades-long melatonin researcher, that we don't know exactly what melatonin is, but we do know what it does.

Dr. Pierpaoli calls melatonin the "master mediator of all hormones" and the "universal chemical mediator of the biological world." He even enthusiastically calls it "the miracle molecule." That's pretty impressive! But does melatonin live up to all the hype? In a single word "Yes."

Among the things we do know:

๛ Like hormones, melatonin is produced in many parts of the body.

🦗 It functions as the body's "aging clock," * It is connected to circadian rhythms, the day-night/sleep-wake cycle, produced by the pineal gland in darkness.

🦗 It is the messenger of the pineal gland, the body's "aging clock" to send a message of youth throughout the body, preventing all of the devastation of aging, Dr. Pierpaoli says.

🦗 It can also be produced by the gut and the retina of the eye.

🦗 It is absorbed through the digestive system from a wide variety of foods, including many fruits, vegetables, grains, nuts, seeds, eggs and fish. No hormone is absorbed through food, which is one of the reasons why melatonin cannot be described as a hormone.

🦗 Melatonin levels reach their peak at puberty and diminish as we age.

🦗 It helps break the stress cycle that can result in a plethora of degenerative diseases associated with aging.

Over the past few decades, there has been an abundance of top-quality research on melatonin, but somehow it has flown under the radar of public awareness. Now it's time to change that.

Immune booster

Let's take a few paragraphs here to delve a bit more deeply into the relationship of melatonin and the immune system and what it means in today's environment.

Let us start by repeating that melatonin is a potent antiviral. As far back as 2013, Italian researchers urged the scientific community to conduct further research on melatonin's potential as a virus fighter.

The immune system is immensely complex. Part of its makeup is an alphabet soup of specialized white blood cells called lymphocytes designed to attack "invaders." These invaders are usually pathogens, like viral, bacterial, parasitic or other microbial infections.

Among these NK or Natural Killer cells. Don't you love that term when we're talking about knocking out possibly deadly infections? NK cells are specialized white blood cells that are the immune system's first line of defense against viral infections and cancer cells.

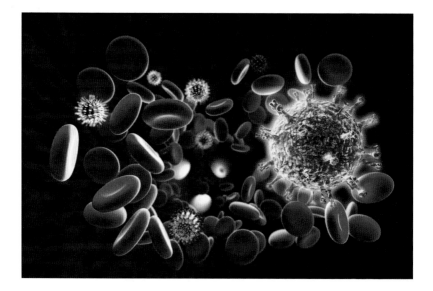

T-cells produced by the thymus gland not only help build a strong immune system, they provide the immune system a power punch to eliminate the infection or the growth of tumor cells. Highly effective T-cells wipe out the infections that the NK cells have attacked. Active and healthy T-cells are essential for survival. With the decline in our number of T-cells as we age, we need something to help us shore up the defenses.

Melatonin is part of the answer, that's for sure.

Melatonin plays a key role in enhancing both of these types of disease-fighting cells. Key 2006 research from a consortium of scientists from around the world confirmed melatonin's role in enhancing the immune system, and says it "has the potential to be useful" in enhancing immune system function and preventing cancerous tumor formation.

What else can melatonin do

Here's a brief list of the scientifically proven effects of melatonin supplements:

CANCER PREVENTION AND TREATMENT: Those immune system boosting T-cells are also the body's primary cancer fighters. By preventing the decline of the immune system as we age, melatonin protects your body from cancer by improving the body's ability to identify and eradicate cells that might turn cancerous. There is also research that shows melatonin is particularly effective in preventing hormonally-related cancers, including breast and prostate cancer.

For those who already have cancer, melatonin has some unique benefits. Researchers from Baylor University found that melatonin overcomes cancer patients' almost inevitable resistance to 5-fluorouracil, a chemotherapy drug often used to treat colorectal and other cancers.

Melatonin helps overcome insomnia, a common side effect of chemotherapy, but, more importantly, melatonin stops the formation of chemoresistant cancer cells. This could be an important advance in cancer treatment and a boon to people with advanced cancers whose options are becoming limited.

HEART HEALTH: Studies show that melatonin reduces artery clogging cholesterol levels, helps keep blood pressure at normal levels and counteracts harmful heart-damaging stress hormones called corticosteroids.

EYE HEALTH: It has been researched and found effective in treating and preventing a variety of eye diseases, including macular degeneration and glaucoma.

GASTROINTESTINAL HEALTH: The GI tract produces 400 times as much melatonin as the pineal gland. Among its powerful effects is giving relief to sufferers from Irritable Bowel Syndrome (IBS) and Inflammatory Bowel Disease (IBD).

CONTROL TYPE 2 DIABETES: It's shown to improve insulin uptake and blood sugar control, especially in older people. It has also been shown to improve the effectiveness of oral anti-diabetes medication as well as preventing some of the more terrible side effects of diabetes, including heart disease and blindness.

TREAT FIBROMYALGIA AND CHRONIC FATIGUE SYNDROME: Studies show melatonin relieved chronic pain in sufferers of both of these disorders and improved quality of life because of better sleep.

SLEEP DISORDERS, OF COURSE: These include insomnia, non 24 sleep/wake disorder, jet lag and sleep disorders caused by pharmaceuticals used for other conditions, including blood pressure.

TREAT INFECTIONS: Clinical data shows that melatonin successfully treats sepsis, a potentially fatal infection in newborns, and herpes viral infections.

WHAT YOU NEED TO KNOW

Melatonin is most commonly used quite effectively for sleep disorders, especially insomnia, but it is little known for its considerable immune system–enhancing effects, including:

- Increasing levels of Natural Killer (NK) cells and T–cells, specialized white blood cells that are at the forefront of infection fighting. Melatonin has been clinically proven to increase the immune system's ability to fight off viral, bacterial, microbial and parasitic infections.

- Boosting immune system enhancing cells, making melatonin a powerful weapon against cancer, especially breast and prostate cancer.

- Effectiveness in preventing and treating:

- Heart disease

- Type 2 diabetes

- Eye diseases like macular degeneration and glaucoma

- Digestive problems including Irritable Bowel Syndrome and Inflammatory Bowel Disease

- Fibromyalgia and chronic fatigue syndrome

- Infections, including the herpes virus and sepsis in newborns

CHAPTER 6

Ramp Up Your
Immune System

In addition to all of its anti-pathogenic effects, andrographis is a
star when it comes to overall immune system enhancement to
prevent infection whenever possible.

In today's world, more is better when it comes to protecting yourself against the onslaught of viruses and other types of
infections. So why not add in the powerhouse of natural immune
boosters?

What a great idea!

SELENIUM

This essential trace mineral boosts immune function by helping lower disease-causing oxidative stress in your body. Studies
show that high blood levels of selenium are especially effective
in strengthening the immune systems of people with influenza,
hepatitis and tuberculosis. Selenium supplements have also been
shown to lead to fewer hospitalizations and an improvement in
symptoms for people who are HIV positive.

A large body of research has shown that selenium helps boost
the immune systems of people with influenza, HIV, tuberculosis
and hepatitis C.

Other research suggests that selenium may stop viruses from
mutating and becoming more virulent and potentially deadly.

Research from Vanderbilt University confirms that 99% of American adults are selenium deficient, giving us at least one explanation for Americans' overall susceptibility to viral and bacterial infections.

Selenium is essential for overall immune function. It works by lowering oxidative stress in your body and reducing inflammation, a major cause of all sorts of chronic diseases.

Low selenium status is associated with greater risk of death from all causes, poor immune function and cognitive decline.

In 2015, Saudi Arabian researchers found that optimal selenium levels decreased the risk of ordinary viruses mutating into deadly pathogens.

What else selenium does

🌰 Science shows that optimal selenium levels lower the risk of several types of cancer, including breast, colon, lung and prostate.

🌰 Reduce risk of heart disease by as much as 50% by reducing the inflammation markers most often associated with heart disease.

🌰 Its antioxidants protect against memory loss, including Parkinson's and Alzheimer's diseases. One interesting small study showed that patients with mild cognitive impairment improved verbal fluency and other mental functions simply by eating just one selenium-rich Brazil nut a day.

🌰 It's essential to proper thyroid function. Thyroid tissue contains more selenium than any other human tissue.

🌰 May improve lung function and help reduce asthma symptoms, again by reducing inflammation.

Best dietary sources of selenium

- Oysters: 238% of the DV in 3 ounces (85 grams)

- Brazil nuts: 174% of the DV in one nut (5 grams)

- Halibut: 171% of the DV in 6 ounces (159 grams)

- Yellowfin tuna: 167% of the DV in 3 ounces (85 grams)

- Eggs: 56% of the DV in 2 large eggs (100 grams)

- Sardines: 46% of the DV in 4 sardines (48 grams)

- Sunflower seeds: 27% of the DV in 1 ounce (28 grams)

- Chicken breast: 12% of the DV in 4 slices (84 grams)

- Shitake mushrooms: 10% of the DV in 1 cup (97 grams

Selenium supplements

Recommended daily intake of selenium supplements for adults is 55–150 mcg of selenium per day. If you are using selenium as a cancer fighter, the recommended daily dosage is 200 mcg.

ZINC

Zinc is an essential mineral vital for immune system function. It is well-known for wound healing.

Hundreds of studies confirm the value of zinc in binding to viruses that cause the common cold, reducing viral load in mucosal membranes and suppressing inflammation.

One important scientific review concluded that zinc lozenges taken within 24 hours of the onset of symptoms reduced the duration of colds by 2.25 days in otherwise healthy people, potentially reducing the opportunity for other infections to take hold.

A 2010 laboratory study showed that zinc proved vital for the immune system from the infection of the SARS-CoV in 2002.

What else zinc does

- Is present in every cell of the human body
- Promotes proper growth in children
- Affects metabolism
- Supports over 300 enzymatic reactions, promoting a healthy gut
- Produces protein
- Is important for the senses of smell and taste

Best dietary sources of zinc

- Oysters: 74 mg in 3 oz
- Beef roast: 7 mg in 3 oz
- Crab: 6.5 mg in 3 oz
- Beef patty: 5.3 mg in 3 oz
- Lobster: 3.4 mg in 3 oz
- Baked beans: 2.9 mg in ½ cup
- Pumpkin seeds: 2.2 mg in 1 oz
- Yogurt: 1.7 mg in 8 oz

Zinc recommended dosage

The recommended dosage is 8 mg daily for adult women and 11 for adult men. Zinc deficiency is rare in the United States, but daily supplementation up to 15 mg daily has been shown to reduce the number of colds. If you are experiencing symptoms of an onset of a cold or other viral infection, 30–75 mg of zinc a day for up to five days will help reduce the duration of the infection if not the symptoms.

In conclusion...

Selenium and zinc are essential minerals that can make the difference between whether you catch an illness or resist it. They:

- Bolster your disease resistance

- Help you recover from colds, flu and other illnesses faster

- Reduce the duration and intensity of upper respiratory infections

- Strengthen you at a cellular level to fight viral and bacterial infections

Viruses are major threats to our health for children and adults alike. They have become harder to control, but it has become easier to be infected with a virus. You can protect yourself easily, every day.

As strong as these ingredients discussed are on their own, a favorite formula of ours is one that combines all of these key ingredients to optimize immune system function.

Look for a formula that contains 300 mg of andrographis, 65 mcg of selenium from yeast, 15 mg of zinc bisglycinate and 5 mg of melatonin. This formula is best when taken 1–2 hours before bedtime.

PART 2

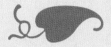

Discover More about Andrographis, the Wonder Healer

CHAPTER 7

Shore Up Liver Function

The liver is the body's most complex organ. It has a role in all metabolic processes in the body. It's the body's storehouse: It converts the fats, carbohydrates and proteins into substances that the body can use, stores these substances and supplies cells with them when they are needed. It's also the body's filtration system: It absorbs toxic substances and converts them into harmless substances or makes sure they are released from the body.

When things go wrong for a variety of reasons, including overuse of alcohol, liver function is compromised. Metabolic, detoxification and storage functions are impaired, over time leading to cirrhosis, a disease that can lead to liver failure, a life-threatening condition.

Milk thistle is a tried and true traditional remedy for all sorts of liver problems, but the ability of andrographis to protect the liver has surpassed even the stellar reputation of milk thistle.

In one study, andrographis has even been shown to cure— completely eliminate—80% of cases of infectious hepatitis, a serious liver disease caused by a variety of viruses.

In another study published in 2014, Taiwanese research shows that andrographis is an effective treatment for hepatitis C, a viral disease that, if untreated, can lead to liver cancer, liver failure and death. The CDC estimates that 3.2 million Americans carry the hepatitis virus, although about half of them don't know it. Researchers theorize that the potent antiviral effects of andrographis are responsible for the successful treatment of this terrible disease.

If you've been paying close attention to Chapters 3 and 4, we are sure you join us in the conclusion that Andrographis is one of the most powerful weapons modern science has against nearly all types of infection we see today, especially viral infections.

WHAT YOU NEED TO KNOW

➤ Andrographis is an effective treatment for liver diseases caused by a variety of viruses, including hepatitis A, B, C, D and E.

➤ Protecting against these viruses can also protect against liver cancer and death from the disease.

CHAPTER 8

The Cancer Warrior

Cancer is a complex disease that develops in many different multistep ways and requires multiple types of treatment.

Andrographis has components that fight cancer in at least five ways (maybe more—new ones are being confirmed frequently!) and has been clinically proven to be effective at slowing, stopping or even eliminating cancer growth in at least eight of the most deadly forms of the disease. That's why we call andrographis the Cancer Warrior.

Cancer killed more than 609,000 Americans in 2018, according to the National Cancer Institute (NCI).

The most common types of cancer in the U.S. are (in descending order, according to estimated new cases in 2018):

- breast
- lung and bronchial
- prostate
- colorectal
- melanoma
- bladder
- non-Hodgkin's lymphoma
- kidney and renal
- endometrial
- leukemia
- pancreatic
- thyroid
- liver

Remember this list. It will become very important in a few pages.

Let's take a brief look at each of the ways andrographis has been scientifically validated for its potent effects against cancer.

About 1.7 million people will be diagnosed with cancer this year. A sobering fact: The NCI says approximately one in three people diagnosed with cancer will die of the disease.

Probably the most impressive review of the pertinent research on andrographis and cancer comes from an international consortium of 19 scientists that confirmed andrographis' anticancer effects "on almost all types of cell lines" by:

🌿 neutralizing free radical damage and inflammation

🌿 stopping out-of-control cell lifespans

🌿 normalizing immune system response

🌿 stopping cells from spreading throughout the body, usually through the bloodstream

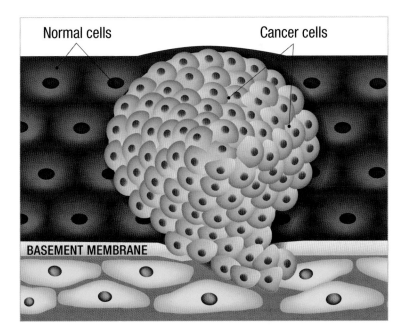

❧ killing cancer-causing cells by forcing them to commit suicide and starving them.

Apoptosis

All cells in the human body have a specific life span, programmed into our DNA. Our cells are living and dying every single day of our lives and each cell is programmed to adhere to that finite lifespan, a biological process called apoptosis. In a strange sequence, chemical messages are sent to the cells telling them quite literally to commit suicide. The DNA of the cells is destroyed by enzymes released as a result of these chemical messages. The cell's surface bubbles away and chemical sweepers usher the dead cells out of the body, but not before they have reproduced themselves.

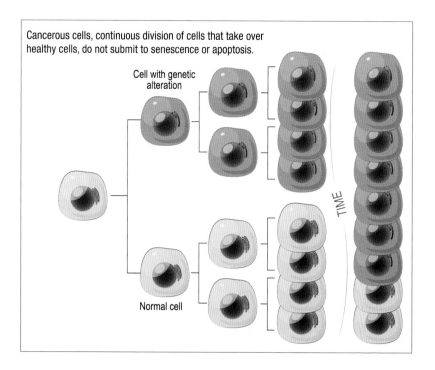

Cancerous cells, continuous division of cells that take over healthy cells, do not submit to senescence or apoptosis.

Cell with genetic alteration

Normal cell

TIME

Healthy red blood cells live for about four months and they are replaced with new cells that are an exact duplicate of parent cells. White blood cells live for a year or more, but skin cells live only two or three weeks; colon cells die after about only four days. The human body replaces an astonishing one million cells per second.

Sometimes things go wrong for reasons not yet fully understood by modern science, when apoptosis fails and cells don't die at the end of their normal lifespan or they do not reproduce exactly the same as parent cells.

With cancer, those immortal cells can continue indefinitely, clump together to form tumors and can eventually kill the patient.

Numerous studies have confirmed that andrographis "wakes up" the body's communication pathways to cells and tells them to return to their normal lifespans.

Andrographis has been confirmed to induce apoptosis in numerous studies confirming this process for several types of cancer, including breast, prostate and colon cancer, and melanoma, a deadly type of skin cancer.

Andrographis literally gets the cells' lifespan back on the right track and wipes out tumors.

Korean research on andrographis confirmed the herb's ability to induce apoptosis in gastric cancers and to slow or even stop the growth of tumors through the actions of other anticancer proteins.

Antioxidant

In the last chapter, we mentioned the antioxidant properties of andrographis. Let's take a moment to look at exactly what that means.

We need oxygen. Without oxygen, you will die in a few minutes. When you breathe in oxygen, oxygen molecules (oxidants) are normally converted into water by your cells. When this conversion is incomplete, so-called "free radicals" are generated. This can happen for many reasons, including insufficient oxygen to the brain (hypoxia), emotional stress, infections, pollution, and toxic exposure, etc. That results in the disease-causing process called oxidative stress.

Those dangerous free radicals generated through oxidative stress cause cellular damage and dysfunction, resulting in disease.

Normal cells have a built-in antioxidant system, which declines with age and becomes unable to neutralize free radicals. This is the underlying cause of many of the diseases of aging, including cancer, heart disease, diabetes and Alzheimer's.

Andrographis is a "strong antioxidant compound," according to Indian research published in 2014 and confirmed by several later studies, including Polish research published in 2015.

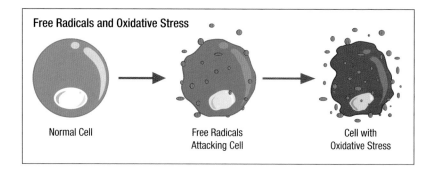

Free Radicals and Oxidative Stress

Normal Cell   Free Radicals   Cell with
             Attacking Cell   Oxidative Stress

Immune booster

As we learned in earlier chapters, andrographis stimulates the immune system, as shown in many studies, largely by activating infection-fighting white blood cells that find and kill bacteria, viruses and other "foreign" substances in the blood.

Small doses of andrographolides, natural bacteria found in the stems and leaves of the andrographis plant, all contribute to the immune boosting effects of the plant. As you know, in higher doses, andrographis calms down immune response and inflammation.

Here's some fairly heavy science, for those who love this sort of thing:

As we've already determined, andrographolides are proven anti-inflammatories. This is especially important in a series of cell-signaling proteins called NF-kB that promote cancer in a variety of ways.

NF-κB is present in almost all human cell types and is activated in response to stress, inflammatory substances, free radicals, heavy metals, ultraviolet irradiation and bacterial or viral infections.

NF-κB also has a vital role in protecting against bacterial and viral infections, however it treads a delicate line. Too much NF-κB is bad because it can turn on genes that tell the cells to divide wildly and stops apoptosis (programmed cell death).

Taiwanese research confirms the value of andrographis in stimulating a very specific anti-inflammatory cell signaling pathway that tells the immune system to fight wild cell division, like we find in cancer.

In the simplest terms, this means that andrographis tells the immune system to control abnormal cell growth.

Angiogenesis

All living beings require nutrients in some form to survive. Cancer cells and cancerous tumors are no different.

Angiogenesis is the process of growing a blood vessel network to nourish a cancerous tumor and allowing it to thrive and grow.

It stands to reason that cutting off that blood supply and oxygen, thus eliminating nutrients, will stop a cancerous tumor from growing and spreading.

Andrographis' ability to cut off the blood supply to tumors is exactly what Chinese researchers were able to confirm with laboratory studies on breast cancer cell lines.

Tumor suppression

Cell damage means damaged DNA, so cells are no longer able to reproduce themselves exactly. This results in the formation of tumors, among other problems.

Chinese researchers found that andrographis stops the cycle of melanoma cancer cell growth. Based on past statistics and the fact that the rate of melanoma has been growing for the past 30 years, the American Cancer Association estimated that over 90,000 Americans were diagnosed with this potentially deadly form of skin cancer in 2018 alone.

Similar results have been seen in studies of pancreatic cancer cells and in glioblastoma cells, an aggressive form of brain cancer.

Brand new results confirm that andrographis in combination with oligomeric proanthocyanidins in French grape seed extract also put a halt to tumor growth in animal studies and on test samples grown from tumors of people with colorectal cancer.

Andrographis has also been shown to stop the growth and formation of pancreatic tumor cells, and limit the ability of glioblastoma cells to migrate. In each study, andrographolide worked along different pathways, showing the versatility of this wonder herb.

Overall, a recent review showed that this one component of andrographis stopped tumor replication in virtually every type of cancer tested and addressed virtually every mechanism, including inflammation, oxidation, cell replication and cancer cell invasion. The authors concluded, "After careful consideration of the relevant evidence, we suggest that andrographolide can be one of the potential agents in the treatment of cancer in the near future."

Enhances conventional cancer therapy

Breaking News: Exciting new research from the City of Hope Medical Center in California confirms that andrographis significantly improves the effectiveness of conventional chemotherapy treatments. Colorectal cancer is notoriously resistant to conventional chemotherapy drugs, like the commonly used 5FU. The research shows that andrographis administered with 5FU improved responses in people with end stage colorectal cancer.

Banishes chemo brain

Andrographis, the cancer warrior, once again comes to the rescue.

"Chemo brain" is a well-documented side effect of chemotherapy used to treat a wide variety of types of cancer. It's characterized by loss of memory, confusion, difficulty concentrating, searching for words, difficulty learning new skills, brain fog and fatigue.

These are almost precisely the symptoms of various forms of dementia.

The Mayo Clinic adds that chemotherapy is probably not the sole cause of chemo brain and that the psychological and physical stress of a cancer diagnosis can contribute to chemo brain. Radiation and other medications associated with cancer treatment may contribute to memory loss and other brain dysfunction for some cancer patients. Most people with chemo brain improve within six to nine months after treatment has ended, but some have long-term memory loss.

Recent German research suggests andrographis may help prevent toxic side effects from chemotherapy and the brain fog or chemo brain that sometimes accompanies conventional cancer treatment. At the same time, andro has been shown to enhance the effectiveness of chemo treatments against cancer cells, meaning lower doses of the drugs may be effective with fewer side effects.

Chinese researchers confirmed that andrographis works synergistically with a commonly prescribed chemotherapy drug for breast cancer (paclitaxel) reducing tumor size by as much as 98%.

A note to those who are working with an oncologist

Don't be surprised if your doctor has never heard of andrographis. Don't be surprised if your oncologist says you shouldn't take it. Please turn to Chapter 13—it's written in more scientific language aimed directly at your doctor. It's probably not realistic to expect your doctor to read this entire book, but we encourage you to copy those few pages. It should be very effective at convincing your doctor about the value of andrographis to treat cancer without interfering with other cancer treatments. You might want to copy the reference section as well.

In conclusion...

Please look back at the beginning of this chapter and the 14 most common cancers in the United States. Andrographis has been scientifically validated to treat every single one of these cancers. It works in at least one way against them and in some cases, it works in multiple ways without interfering with conventional cancer treatment. Since there are no serious side effects from using andrographis, it's really an obvious course of action for anyone who has been diagnosed with cancer.

WHAT YOU NEED TO KNOW

Andrographis addresses cancer in at least five ways, possibly more, by:

🥀 normalizing immune system response

🥀 neutralizing free radical damage and inflammation

🥀 stopping out-of-control cell lifespans

🥀 stopping cells from spreading throughout the body, usually in the bloodstream

🥀 killing cancer-causing cells by forcing them to commit suicide, and starving them.

Plus, it relieves side effects of conventional cancer treatment, especially cognitive dysfunction commonly known as "chemo brain."

CHAPTER 9

The Prince of Hearts

Androgeraphis has impressive powers to protect heart health and even to contain damage if you've had a heart attack or stroke, or you have diabetes and you're at high risk for heart problems.

Since heart disease is the Number 1 killer in the Western world, it's worth taking a close look at the benefits of androgeraphis to help reverse that grim statistic.

In the United States, someone dies of cardiovascular disease every 40 seconds. That's 800,000 people every year. Additionally, someone has a stroke every 40 seconds in the US. While death rates from strokes have declined, large numbers of stroke survivors suffer from long-term disability.

Androgeraphis works in a variety of ways to heal and protect the heart and the cardiovascular system. Plus, it's powerful medicine against diabetes. Diabetes is a sinister disease with a multitude of side effects, including heart disease. Many doctors treat people with diabetes as if they've already had a heart attack since the risk is so high. More than 100 million Americans had diabetes or pre-diabetes in 2017, according to the Centers for Disease Control and Prevention.

Read on, friends.

Metabolic syndrome

In recent years, metabolic syndrome, literally a basket of medical problems, has been identified as a red flag for heart disease and diabetes.

Metabolic syndrome has four major characteristics:

- high blood pressure

- high blood fats (cholesterol and triglycerides)

- high blood sugars

- excess abdominal fat

Andrographis offers an answer to all of these, especially the problem of obesity, preventing diabetes and heart disease even when lab animals were fed a high fat diet, according to a joint study by Taiwanese and Indian researchers.

Another team of researchers from Brazil and Bangladesh found that andrographis is effective in treating and preventing cardiovascular disease and diabetes stemming from metabolic syndrome, calling andrographis a "new hope" in the treatment of metabolic syndrome.

Andrographis can be powerful medicine even for those who have only one component of the metabolic syndrome basket of disorders.

Control cholesterol and triglycerides

Research shows that andrographis controls the buildup of artery clogging cholesterol, stops artery-blocking blood clots and directly lowers cholesterol levels.

Taiwanese researchers found that andrographis helps lower fatty accumulations in artery-clogging foam cells, reducing the risk of atherosclerosis, commonly known as hardening of the arteries.

Additionally, a 2015 clinical trial found that andrographis extract was just as effective as gemfibrozil, a pharmaceutical that reduces the amounts of fat produced by the liver in patients with elevated triglycerides (blood fats) and cholesterol. Researchers suggested andrographis might be used as an alternative medicine for high triglycerides. Gemfibrozil can have serious side effects, including muscle weakness, blurred vision, irregular heartbeat and fatigue. Andrographis has no serious side effects.

Lower blood pressure

Anyone who has heart disease, knows anyone with heart disease or is over 40 knows that high blood pressure triggers heart attacks and strokes.

Conventional doctors are rightly focused on controlling blood pressure through diet and medication. Little do most of them know that the answer to hypertension (high blood pressure) is easily available.

Andrographis is a vasorelaxant. That means it helps relax constricted blood vessels, easing the flow of blood and lowering blood pressure.

Our research confirms the abilities of andrographis and andrographolides to lower blood pressure, particularly systolic pressure (the upper number), which is the most dangerous if it's too high.

Furthermore, Armenian and Swedish researchers demonstrated that andrographolides reduce blood clotting in arteries without thinning blood, suggesting beneficial effects on cardiovascular health, blood vessels and prevention of strokes, even though it is not a blood thinner and doesn't require dietary restrictions or expose you to excess bleeding like pharmaceuticals prescribed to reduce clotting.

Beat diabetes

The American Diabetes Association reports that 30.3 million Americans or 9.4% of the population have Type 2 diabetes, the type that usually develops as waistlines increase. About one-third of the people with the disease do not know they have diabetes, increasing their risk of serious side effects including heart attacks and strokes.

One study shows that andrographis reduces blood sugars in diabetic rats by as much as 52.9%.

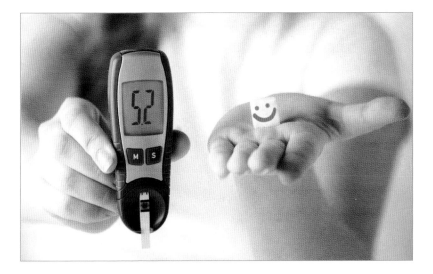

Malaysian researchers found that andrographis was a valuable tool in the treatment of type 1 diabetes (insulin-dependent from the beginning, caused by a failure of the pancreas to produce blood sugar-balancing insulin) and Type 2 diabetes (once called adult onset diabetes, characterized by the body's inability to use the insulin the body produces). This study concluded that andrographis "was found to be quite effective in restoring the disturbed metabolic profile of obese diabetic rats back towards normal conditions."

Control obesity

Non-alcoholic fatty liver disease (NAFLD), largely linked to obesity, affects 80 to 100 million people worldwide, most of them in industrialized countries. More distressing, 25% of American adults (50 million people) have NAFLD, according to the American Liver Foundation. Even more distressing, National Institutes of Health researchers estimate that about 10% of American children ages 2–19 have the condition.

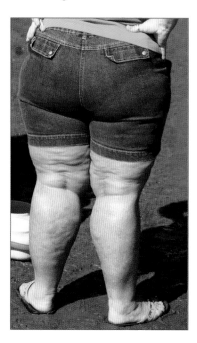

Andrographis to the rescue, again!

Indian research shows the wonder herb lowers the lipids (fats) in the liver effectively without serious side effects.

Obesity is a major risk factor in cardiovascular disease and diabetes.

Exciting research from a Taiwanese team published in early 2020 confirms that andrographis is an important tool in the fight against heart disease in obese patients. The animal study showed that andrographis protected their hearts from damage and treated heart damage in obese mice, even when they were fed a high-fat diet.

An even more exciting benefit of andrographis...

As far back as 1991, researchers found that administering andrographis within an hour of a heart attack (myocardial infarction) limited damage to the heart and blood vessels, plus it prevented the formation of further clots that could cause another heart attack or stroke. Several studies have since confirmed those early results.

In conclusion...

For decades, researchers have told us of the impressive effects of andrographis in treating and preventing two of the most dangerous diseases known to humankind. For millennia, traditional Asian medicine has known of the value of this Asian herb. Now we "modern" consumers are finally getting on the andrographis bandwagon. It's about time.

WHAT YOU NEED TO KNOW

Andrographis addresses all of the conditions that lead to heart disease, heart attacks, strokes and diabetes:

⟫ it controls high blood pressure

⟫ it reduces cholesterol and blood fats (triglycerides)

⟫ it reduces the risk of diabetes, which puts its victims at high risk for heart disease

⟫ it limits the basket of risk factors known as metabolic syndrome that contribute to increased risk of heart disease and diabetes.

CHAPTER 10

The Energy Wizard

If you are over 50, I imagine you have complained at least once that your memory is not as sharp as it once was or that you wish you had the energy you had when you were 30, or that stress seems to be frying your brain. Does that sound familiar?

There is a unique phenomenon in human physiology called the blood brain barrier or BBB. It's a mechanism that protects the brain and spinal fluid by preventing most substances from passing into the brain through the capillaries (the smallest blood vessels).

Andrographis is one of the few substances that can cross the BBB, giving it unique access to the brain and to healing where it is needed, especially when you are overstressed, low in energy, worried about fading memory or even specific brain impairment.

What's more, when andrographolides cross into the brain, they concentrate there and in the spinal cord, prolonging their effect.

Remember when we talked about adaptogens in Chapter 2? The considerable powers of andrographis to bring about homeostasis or physiological balance—are particularly evident when we're talking about energy and emotional and brain health.

Stress

It's impossible to be alive in today's world without psychological and physical stress and to survive without an ability to adapt to severe stress.

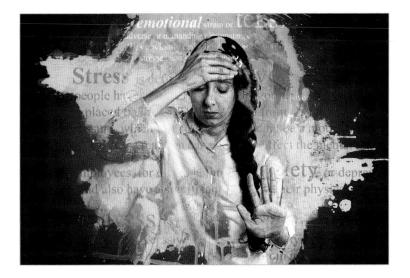

We all experience the daily emotional stresses of traffic jams, job pressure, relationship challenges and more. What's more important is how we cope with stress and even severe stress levels—Dr. Panossian calls it dis-stress—and its destructive effects on us.

Physical stressors are sometimes less noticeable than emotional stressors. The subtle changes in cellular structure and even DNA caused by omnipresent chemical pollutants as well as increasingly intense weather and temperature fluctuations, cigarette smoke, over processed foods and overmedication can have profound effects on our health.

The combination of physical and emotional stress can be devastating and even deadly.

Given the adaptogenic nature of andrographis, it's not surprising that a substantial amount of research confirms the herb's ability to help us manage both types of stress.

One Indian study shows that andrographis is much more effective than diazepam (Valium) in lab animals exposed to stressful conditions. And a 2014 study from India confirmed that andrographis, even at low doses, relieved the symptoms of long-term stress and lowered levels of the stress hormone cortisol.

Energy

Hand-in-hand with the unrelieved stress that seems to characterize modern life, we often feel sapped. Sleep disturbances prevent us from reaching deep levels of energy-restoring sleep. When you lie awake at night reliving the events of the day or anticipating the events of coming days, you don't get the restorative sleep you need to renew energy levels and brain function.

If you wake up still tired and even more stressed, we've got an answer for you.

You guessed it! Take andrographis!

A 2016 Chilean study of patients with multiple sclerosis, an energy-sapping autoimmune disease characterized by inflammation and nerve deterioration, experienced a dramatic increase in their energy levels after taking andrographis.

Using an assessment tool called the Fatigue Severity Score, patients in the study reported they were 44% less fatigued after taking andrographis for a year. As a bonus, researchers theorized, the anti-inflammatory effects of andrographis also reduced scarring on the nerve fibers, moderating the effects of the disease.

Memory and dementia

More than almost anything else, many of us fear loss of memory in old age.

In the United States, one in 10 people over 65 has Alzheimer's disease. Two-thirds of the victims of the memory-destroying disease are women. Most disturbing is the fact reported by the Alzheimer's Association that deaths from the disease increased by 123% between 2000 and 2015, at the same time that deaths from all other diseases declined significantly.

The prevalence of Alzheimer's disease in India and China is much lower than in the rest of the Western world at 4.86%. That certainly means we have something to learn from our Asian friends.

Scientists offer a variety of reasons why Indian and Chinese people have some sort of protections, but we'll venture a guess that andrographis has a role since it is so widely used in both countries' traditional medicines and, as you'll see in the coming paragraphs, research has confirmed andrographis' value in preventing and treating Alzheimer's.

In India, we'll also venture to guess, the presence of curcumin in curry dishes consumed on a daily basis for a lifetime contributes

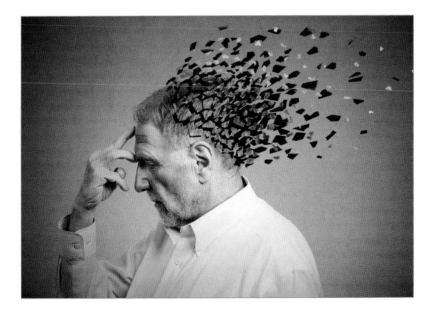

to some form of protection against dementia. Curcumin is well studied for its effectiveness against Alzheimer's disease.

Our most recent research published in the journal *Pharmaceuticals* confirms Andro's effectiveness against memory loss in humans with mild memory impairment. There aren't many human or clinical trials that are randomized, double-blind and placebo-controlled, two-armed crossover studies—the gold standard of scientific research, so the results were really impressive. It's now scientifically confirmed that andrographis can be used as effective and safe treatment for impaired cognitive function, memory, learning abilities and sleep disorders without making subjects sleepy.

Perhaps the most comprehensive study on andrographis and Alzheimer's disease came from Chilean scientists, published in 2016 in the journal *Neurobiology of Aging*. Using a unique breed of wild South American rodents with a tendency to develop Alzheimer's with age, they discovered that andrographis not only worked to prevent Alzheimer's, it actually helped reverse memory loss.

The Chilean study confirmed that andrographis works in at least four ways to preserve and restore cognitive function:

- It helps regain learning performance and spatial memory (like that used to navigate through a familiar neighborhood or city).

- It helps restore the ability of brain cells to communicate with each other.

- It protects vital proteins to maintain and preserve the chemical and electrical communication systems within the brain.

- It protects the neurons, the brain cells that are at the core of all thought and memory processes.

Even more impressive, an Indian-German collaboration published in early 2018, concludes that andrographis protects the brains of laboratory animals with diabetes. Since people with diabetes are at high risk of Alzheimer's disease, the scientists concluded that the Ayurvedic herb may be a useful tool to help protect the brains of people with diabetes. Alzheimer's disease has sometimes been called Type 3 diabetes.

In conclusion

Overall, the actions of andrographis—addressing our stress and stressors and our adaptability to challenges, helping brain cells communicate more clearly and boosting energy levels—makes it an excellent adaptogenic herb and treatment for stress, fatigue and cognitive dysfunction.

WHAT YOU NEED TO KNOW

Andrographis works in a variety of ways to:

- Relieve long-term physical and emotional stress-induced damage, reducing the risk of a wide variety of the diseases of aging that have been directly linked to unrelieved stress.

- Help regain energy and dramatically reduce fatigue, even in people who have serious chronic diseases.

- Cross the blood-brain barrier and work in very specific ways to protect brain cells and even to restore brain function in people with Alzheimer's disease and other forms of dementia.

CHAPTER 11

And a Whole Lot More...

If you haven't heard enough about the powers of the King of Bitters, there is more, much more.

Preventing and treating cancer, HIV/AIDS, heart disease and more are impressive properties, so why not add in another laundry list of study-proven benefits of this impressive herb?

Andrographis has been confirmed as a treatment and or preventive for:

- digestive issues
- ulcerative colitis
- colic
- gallstones

- malaria
- snakebite
- infertility
- maybe even hangovers...

We're the first to admit this a mixed bag of conditions that don't seem to have any connection. When Dr. Panossian first began researching andrographis, he was just as surprised by its powers as we are sure you are.

Digestive issues

Andrographis has been proven to be an effective treatment for a wide variety of digestive issues.

General indigestion

Bitter herbs have long been used to address that general tummy ache, heartburn, bloating, belching and flatulence. What better way to address those everyday problems than with andrographis, the King of Bitters?

The bitter taste on your tongue stimulates the production of saliva, the first stage of digestion.

Bitters promote healthy digestion by stimulating the production of stomach acid, bile and digestive enzymes that help break down food and make the nutrients available to your body.

Colic

If you've ever had a screaming infant who won't be comforted, you've entered the world of colic.

Experts don't know the precise cause of this pain that as many as one in four infants experience from birth to the age of about four months. They suggest it may be the result of an underdeveloped digestive system, gas, imbalances of the biome or food intolerances.

Whatever the cause of this anxiety-producing condition for parents and child, andrographis has an answer. No one knows for sure why, but parents in India and Asia have found andrographis is a godsend for colicky babies.

Gallbladder

The gallbladder is connected to the liver and intestines by ducts that transport bile, the "detergents" of the digestive system that help break down fats.

Animal studies show that andrographis increased bile production, improved gallbladder function, improved fat metabolism and prevented the formation of gallstones.

Diarrhea

Diseases that cause diarrhea are numerous, but especially for children, diarrhea itself is a leading cause of death in the developing world. One impressive Chinese study published in 1993 showed that andrographis treatment coupled with a rehydration regimen for six days cured E. coli infections in 82.5% of the patients in the study and is as effective as commonly prescribed antidiarrheal drugs.

Ulcerative colitis

This painful condition is an inflammatory bowel disease that causes inflammation and ulcers (sores) inside the digestive tract, most often in the colon. People with ulcerative colitis (UC) experience severe diarrhea, abdominal pain, urgency to defecate, weight loss, fatigue, fevers and more. Ulcerative colitis usually develops slowly and patients who are correctly treated can go into remission. UC is not curable, but it is manageable.

Andrographis appears to be a safe way to treat UC, according to researchers from the University of California at La Jolla who studied the effects of the Ayurvedic herb on more than 200 patients with mild to moderate UC. They found that 60% of their patients achieved remission within eight weeks at a dosage of 1,800 mg of unstandardized andrographis daily. Lower amounts are just as effective in standardized products.

Malaria

The best guess of scientists is that there are 219 million cases of malaria around the world every year resulting in about 435,000 deaths, more than 90% of them in African countries.

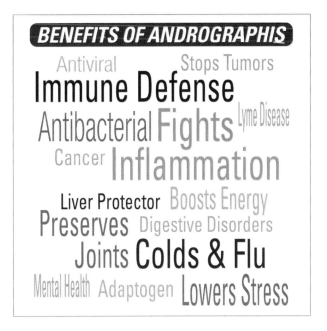

Malaria is caused by a parasite carried by infected female mosquitoes.

The malaria death rate has been reduced by approximately 50% since 2000, largely because of widespread insecticide spraying and the distribution of insecticide infused mosquito nets in Africa, although there are obvious and well-documented negative effects of prolonged exposure to insecticides.

The multi-tasking antimicrobial powers of andrographis to the rescue once again!

At least four studies confirm the benefits of four specific andrographolides against the parasites that cause malaria.

An Indian study published in 2009 also confirmed that andrographis inhibited at least half of the active parasites. The effects were even more powerful when andrographis was combined with curcumin.

Snakebite

Fortunately, we don't have cobras in the Western world, but if we did, we'd embrace the findings that andrographis can combat even the world's most deadly snake venom that claims as many as 50,000 lives a year in India alone.

Andrographis has traditionally been administered after a cobra bite, which paralyzes the breathing apparatus and is almost always fatal within 24 hours. This is especially important in rural areas where hospitals and more modern treatment modalities are not readily available, and may help keep victims alive until they can get to a hospital.

ANDROGRAPHIS
The Answer for Optimal Health

Preserves Cognitive Health: Andrographis has adaptogenic effects that help you stay resilient in the face of stress, and helps brain cells communicate better.

Protects Heart and Arteries: Andrographis stops arterial blockage and relaxes blood vessels to keep your blood pressure healthy and prevent cardiovascular damage.

Protects the Liver: Andrographis has been traditionally recommended to help the liver detoxify and to repair damage to the liver by improving levels of the body's own natural antioxidants.

Stops Pain, Preserves Joints: Andrographis directly inhibits pain-causing COX-2 activity, and protects the cushioning cartilage between joints.

Stops or Prevents Tumors: Scientific research shows that this powerful botanical stops DNA damage and the development and proliferation of brain, skin, and pancreatic cancer cells.

Boosts Immune Defenses: This herb has been shown in clinical studies to reduce cold and flu symptoms. It also fights dangerous, drug-resistant bacteria and can even stop Lyme disease.

Soothes Digestive Symptoms: Andrographis balances pH levels in the stomach, stops inflammation associated with ulcerative colitis, and protects the lining of stomach and intestines against ulcers.

An Indian lab study showed that about one-third of animals survived when they were administered andrographis after they were given snake venom. None survived without andrographis.

Hangover

We're probably going back to the liver stimulation and protective properties of andrographis when we find clinical evidence that the miracle herb can cure a hangover.

It's been used traditionally and is mentioned in at least one study published in *Current Drug Abuse Reviews* in 2010.

If you've overindulged, it's probably best to drink a lot of water, but adding a capsule of andrographis certainly won't hurt and it may help.

In conclusion...

As we've seen from the earlier chapters of this book, andrographis and its primary beneficial component, andrographolide, is a versatile medicinal to prevent and treat a wide variety of conditions.

This chapter confirms andrographis' pharmacopeia against such widely diverse diseases and conditions as liver dysfunction, digestive issues, including serious ones like ulcerative colitis and more. Its value as a traditional herbal treatment is confirmed by modern research substantiating its curative powers against malaria, snakebite and even possibly for natural birth control.

WHAT YOU NEED TO KNOW

Andrographis has been the subject of broad research that confirms its value for:

❧ Effectively addressing a variety of digestive disorders including inflammatory bowel disease, ulcerative colitis, gallbladder disease, diarrhea, colic and more

❧ Treating malaria, a major cause of death in tropical countries, especially in Africa

❧ Prolonging life after a deadly snake bite until medical attention can be obtained

❧ Relieving hangovers

CHAPTER 12

Know How to Make the Right Choice

From Terry Lemerond

I n the supplement world, there are often confusing choices that serve little purpose except to overwhelm you. I'll try to make the buying decision as simple as possible for you.

How much to take?

Andrographis was brought to my attention by an Indian scientist while I was on a visit to India researching Ayurvedic medicine.

To learn more, I teamed up with Dr. Panossian, who is based in Sweden. He's an expert in botanical medicine, especially adaptogens. He researched andrographis for many years while he was at the Swedish Herbal Institute.

Working together, we discovered some powerful effects when combining andrographis with zinc, selenium and melatonin for a variety of diseases.

Here is my personal formula that I swear by for modulating and strengthening the immune system. I have recommended it to hundreds of people via my radio show and weekly newsletter with very effective results. I think it will make your immune system much healthier and protect you against many diseases as well as viral and upper respiratory tract infections.

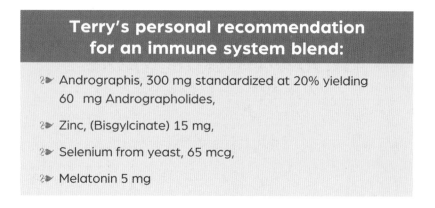

Terry's personal recommendation for an immune system blend:

⮞ Andrographis, 300 mg standardized at 20% yielding 60 mg Andrographolides,

⮞ Zinc, (Bisgylcinate) 15 mg,

⮞ Selenium from yeast, 65 mcg,

⮞ Melatonin 5 mg

Keep in mind melatonin works only at night, so the only time I suggest taking this combination is 60–90 minutes before bed time. You can take the above blend 1–4 times nightly.

Look for this formula in a capsule form, and take 1–4 capsules before bedtime.

You may be thinking you don't need melatonin to sleep. Neither do I, but I find I sleep more soundly and wake up much more refreshed when I take it.

I have spent the last year researching melatonin.

I found there are 24,500 studies, (no, I did not read all of them!) but from the hundreds I reviewed on cancer, upper respiratory viral infections, anti-aging benefits or heart disease, I realized melatonin is a very effective and powerful molecule that could possibly be the master regulator of all body functions.

Yes, it does help immensely as a sleep agent, but there would never have been 24,500 studies on melatonin if that's all it did.

But everyone should follow their gut feeling, and if melatonin is just NOT for you, then I suggest taking andrographis on its own.

I think you'll get the best results with 400 mg of andrographis standardized at 20% andrographolides 1–3 times daily.

These levels or even higher are effective for the spectrum of health conditions that Dr. Panossian and I have addressed in this book.

As always, consult a knowledgeable medical professional, especially if you are addressing cancer, heart disease or dementia with andrographis. If your doctor is not familiar with andrographis or reflexively says you shouldn't take it, please copy Chapter 13 of this book and entreat your doctor to spend a few minutes reading it.

Some people choose to take andrographis on a temporary basis for seven to ten days to treat colds or flu or other acute infections. Others take it for years on end to treat serious health issues such as cancer or heart disease, or cognitive dysfunction with no apparent negative effects. You can safely take 1 to 4 times the recommended dosages if you have serious health conditions like these.

The most frequently reported side effect was a mild skin rash that disappeared as soon as people stopped taking the herb.

Anaphylaxis, a severe and life-threatening allergic reaction, has been reported in a handful of people taking andrographis in very high dosages, over 5 grams daily.

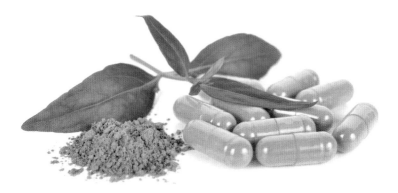

CHAPTER 13

Doc-to-Doc:
How Andrographis
Can Help Your Patients

From Dr. Panossian

Dear Doctor:

Like most books, this book is copyrighted. However, the information presented here is so important to your patients' health and to your scientific knowledge that we have urged ours readers to copy this chapter and give it to you in hope that this brief summary of efficacy of *andrographis paniculata* will help you recognize its effectiveness in preventing and treating a broad spectrum of disease conditions.

First, let me briefly introduce myself:

I am Alexander Panossian, Ph.D. and Dr. Sci. in bioorganic chemistry, the chemistry of natural and physiologically active compounds. I have been a professor in this discipline since 1991, working in Sweden since 2003 at the Swedish Herbal Institute and as a founder of Phytomed AB in Sweden. I was editor-in-chief of Phytomedicine, an international journal of phytotherapy and phytopharmacology from 2014-2017. I have been credited as lead researcher or participant in more than 180 articles published in peer-reviewed journals, and I hold four US patents. My major interest is in plant adaptogens.

I enthusiastically support the use of andrographis for a wide variety of conditions, as delineated below. I strongly urge you to consider andrographis not only for colds and flu, as it is most commonly used, but for other infectious and inflammatory diseases, immunomodulation, cell life cycle modulation, hepatoprotection, neurodegenerative impairment and metabolic disorders.

Andrographolides, the major active ingredients in andrographis, are diterpenoid lactones—rare compounds with strong anti-inflammatory, antioxidant and antimicrobial effects. Andrographis is also a rich source of other biologically active compounds, including well-researched antioxidant polyphenols.

Andrographis has been used for centuries in Traditional Chinese Medicine and Ayurvedic medicine and is revered for its adaptogenic effects.

The abbreviated information I am about to present to you is substantiated by hundreds of peer-reviewed studies. I am attaching citations to a few major reviews at the end of this chapter. If you would like further references, please ask the patient who gave this piece to you to copy the reference section of this book.

List of conditions for which andrographis has been well-researched:

- all types of viral infections

- colds, flu, upper respiratory infections: prevents infection and shortens duration

- joint pain, arthritis

- infection fighting, including staph, salmonella and MRSA

- liver disease

- Lyme disease

- pneumococcal pneumonia, including antibiotic resistant strains
- cancer: almost all types
- virus fighting, including the herpes simplex virus
- malaria and other illnesses caused by parasites
- ulcerative colitis and other digestive problems
- multiple sclerosis
- Alzheimer's disease and dementia
- heart disease by lowering cholesterol and blood pressure, dissolving blood clots
- diabetes, types 1 and 2
- rheumatoid arthritis and other autoimmune diseases

Andrographis has been shown to be as effective as pharmaceuticals in many cases, and sometimes even more effective, without serious side effects. Rare reports of anaphylaxis have been reported in patients taking very high amounts, far above the recommended dosage.

Multifaceted Andrographis

ANTI-INFECTIOUS: Through multiple studies, andrographis has been confirmed as antiviral, antibacterial, antifungal and antiparasitic. It is most commonly used to prevent and treat colds and flu and has been shown to dramatically reduce the duration of colds and flu. Research substantiates andrographis stops the herpes virus from entering cells. It has been found to be an effective adjunct to conventional therapies for HIV/AIDS. It's also been used successfully against antibiotic resistant Staphylococcus aureus bacteria and MRSA.

IMMUNOMODULATION: The adaptogenic effects of andrographis (adaptogens promote homeostasis) successfully treat allergies and allergic asthma and a variety of autoimmune diseases

ANTI-INFLAMMATORY: Andrographis has been researched to successfully treat a wide variety of chronic inflammatory conditions, including arthritis and joint pain, allergies and allergic asthma

NEURODEGENERATIVE IMPAIRMENT: Inflammation is the common thread of Alzheimer's, dementia, Parkinson's and multiple sclerosis. Research confirms that andrographis can prevent nerve deterioration, help recover memory (in animal studies) and reduce

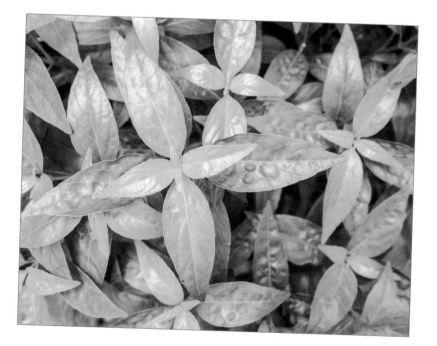

fatigue in MS patients. It also significantly reduced inflammatory factors that worsen Parkinson's.

CELL LIFE CYCLE MODULATION: In vivo and in vitro studies confirm that andrographis induces apoptosis, inhibits angiogenesis, suppresses tumors, suppresses oxidative stress by neutralizing free radical damage and enhances immune function, making it an effective tool against a wide variety of cancers, including breast, colon, brain and pancreatic. It has also been shown to reduce the brain fog often associated with chemotherapy.

METABOLIC DISORDERS: Andrographis has been shown to be effective at controlling the various factors of metabolic syndrome that lead to diabetes and heart disease, including controlling blood pressure, lipids, blood sugars and excess abdominal fat.

CARDIOPROTECTIVE: The above factors are, of course, helpful in controlling cardiovascular disease, especially its antihypertensive and antilipidemic effects. Andrographis has also been shown to inhibit platelet aggregation.

HEPATOPROTECTIVE: Andrographis has been shown to cure —completely eradicate—80% of infectious hepatitis and it has been shown effective against hepatitis C, probably because of its antiviral properties. A 2014 Malaysian study concluded, "The standardized extract of A. paniculata with the right phytochemical composition of diterpenic labdanes is likely to have tremendous potential for the development of hepatoprotective medicine. This standardized herbal medicine may not provide immediate remedy, but it can be considered as a comprehensive therapy for liver inflammation.

DIGESTIVE ISSUES: Andrographis is a bitter herb, so it is an effective medicinal for a variety of digestive issues, including general indigestion, colic, gallbladder disease and gallstones, diarrhea and inflammatory bowel disease, including ulcerative colitis.

There's more...

Malaria

Andrographis' anti-parasitic effects are credited for its effectiveness against malaria. At least four studies confirm the benefits of four specific andrographolides against the parasites that cause malaria. An Indian study published in 2009 also confirmed that andrographis inhibited at least half of the active parasites and the effects were even more powerful when andrographis was combined with curcumin.

Similar properties are the likely explanation for andrographis' efficacy against Lyme disease as well.

Snakebite

Andrographis has traditionally been used after a cobra bite, which paralyzes the breathing apparatus and is almost always fatal within 24 hours. This is especially important in rural areas where hospitals and more modern treatment modalities are not readily available, and may help keep victims alive until they can get to a hospital.

Safety

Products containing *andrographis paniculata* have been found safe during the clinical studies in adults.

The safety of products containing andrographis has not been evaluated in children and adolescents.

The safety of use during pregnancy and lactation has not been reliably studied.

In conclusion...

I recommend 300 mg of andrographis extract standardized to 20% for a total of 60 mg of andrographolide one or two times daily for most of these conditions.

Research has shown that a total of 1,200 mg of andrographis extract daily resulted in no changes in liver or kidney function, blood counts or other laboratory measures. One review of all clinical reports of adverse events resulting from treatment of upper respiratory tract infections with *andrographis paniculata* found only "mild, infrequent and reversible adverse events. The most frequent ones included pruritus, fatigue, headache and diarrhea."

A substantial body of research suggests that adding melatonin (up to 10 mg daily) significantly improves immune function and contains potent antiviral properties

The addition of selenium (65–200 mcg from yeast), zinc bis-glycinate (15–60 mg) and melatonin (5–20 mg) all have validated potentiation.

I have studied andrographis in my laboratory for more than 20 years and I find it to be highly efficacious. I hope you will consider it as well.

—Alexander Panossian, Ph.D., Dr. Sci.

Reviews of Andrographis*

Panossian A. Evolution of Adaptogenic Concept: New Evidence on Potential Use of Adaptogens in Stress-Induced and Aging-Related disorders. 22nd International Congress Phytochemicals in Medicine and Food. 25–27 June 2018, Horgen and ZHAW Wadenswil, Switzerland.

Panossian A. Wikman G. Efficacy of Andrographis paniculata in upper respiratory tract (URT) infectious diseases and the mechanism of action. In: Evidence and rational based research on Chinese Drugs, Ed. H. Wagner and G. Ulrich Merzenich (Eds.), Springer Publ. Comp. 2012. Pp. 137–180.

Assessment report on Andrographis paniculata Nees, folium. 27 August 2014 EMA/HMPC/320433/2012 Corr1 Committee on Herbal Medicinal Products (HMPC)

Herba Andrographidis, 2002. WHO Monographs on Selected Medicinal Plants, vol. 2. WHO, Geneva, pp.12–242002.

Hossain MS, Urbi Z et al. Andrographis paniculata (Burm. F.) Wall ex Nees: A Review of Ethnobotany, phytochemistry and Pharmacology. The Scientific World Journal;2014 274905.

Dai Y, Chen SR et al. Overview of pharmacological activities of Andrographis paniculata and its major compound andrographolide. Crit Rev Food Sci Nutr. 2018 Sep 10:1–13.

Hu XY, Wu RH et al. Andrographis paniculata (Chuan Xin Lian) for symptomatic relief of acute respiratory infections in adults and children: A systematic review and meta-analysis. PLos One, 2017 Aug 4;12(8):e0181780.

Islam MT, Ali ES, et al., Andrographolide, a diterpene

lactone from Andrographis paniculata and its therapeutic promises in cancer. Cancer Lett. 2018 Apr 28;420:129–145

Islam MT. Andrographolide, a New Hope in the Prevention and Treatment of Metabolic Syndrome. Front Pharmacol. 2017 Aug 23;8:571.

Tan WSD, Liao W, Zhou S, Wong WSF. Is there a future for andrographolide to be an anti-inflammatory drug? Deciphering its major mechanisms of action. Biochem Pharmacol. 2017 Sep 1;139:71–81.

Akbar S. Andrographis paniculata: a review of pharmacological activities and clinical effects. Altern Med Rev. 2011 Mar;16(1):66-77.

* A more detailed accounting of andrographis research is contained in the entire book *The Wonders of Andrographis* by Alexander Panossian, available on Amazon.

References

REVIEWS

Akbar, S. 2011. Andrographis paniculata: a review of pharmacological activities and clinical effects. Altern Med Rev. 16, 66–77.

Assessment report on andrographis paniculata Nees, folium. 27 August 2014 EMA/HMPC/320433/2012 Corr1 Committee on Herbal Medicinal Products (HMPC)

Dai, Y., Chen, S.R. et al. 2018. Overview of pharmacological activities of andrographis paniculata and its major compound andrographolide. Crit Rev Food Sci Nutr. 10, 1–13.

Herba Andrographidis, 2002. WHO Monographs on Selected Medicinal Plants, vol. 2. WHO, Geneva, pp.12–242002.

Hossain, M.S., Urbi, Z. et al. 2014. Andrographis paniculata (Burm. F.) Wall ex Nees: A Review of Ethnobotany, phytochemistry and Pharmacology. The Scientific World Journal. 274905.

Islam, M.T. 2017. Andrographolide, a New Hope in the Prevention and Treatment of Metabolic Syndrome. Front Pharmacol. 8:571.

Islam, M.T., Ali, E.S., et al. 2018. Andrographolide, a diterpenelactone from andrographis paniculata and its therapeutic promises in cancer. Cancer Lett. 420,129–145

Jayakumar, T., Hsieh, C.Y. et al. 2013. Experimental and Clinical Pharmacology of andrographis paniculata and Its Major Bioactive Phytoconstituent Andrographolide. Evid Based Complement Alternat Med. 2013:846740.

Mathuranath, P.S., George, A. et al. 2012. Incidence of Alzheimer's disease in India: a 10 years follow-up study. Neural. India 60,625–630.

Panossian, A., Wikman, G. 2012. Efficacy of andrographis paniculata in upper respiratory tract (URT) infectious diseases and the mechanism of action. In: Evidence and rational based research on Chinese Drugs, Ed. H. Wagner and G. Ulrich Merzenich (Eds.), Springer Publ. Comp. Pp. 137–180.

Panossian, A.G. 1917. Understanding adaptogenic activity: specificity of the pharmacological action of adaptogens and other phytochemicals. Ann. N.Y. Acad. Sci. 1401, 49–64. Full text free access.

Tan, W.S.D., Liao, W., Zhou, S., Wong, W.S.F. 2017. Is there a future for andrographolide to be an anti-inflammatory drug? Deciphering its major mechanisms of action. Biochem Pharmacol.139,71–81.

ORIGINAL STUDIES
Ch 2: Andrographis : The King of Bitters

Panossian, A., Kochikian A. et al. 1999. Effect of andrographis panicuiata extract on progesterone in blood plasma of pregnant rats. Phytomedicine. 6,157–162.

Panossian, A., Seo, E.J., Efferth, T. 2018. Novel molecular mechanisms for the adaptogenic effects of herbal extracts on isolated brain cells using systems biology. Phytomedicine 50, 257–284.

Suriyo, T., Pholpana, N. et al. 2017. Clinical Parameters following Multiple Oral Dose Administration of a Standardized Andrographis paniculata Capsule in Healthy Thai Subjects. Planta Med. 83, 778–789.

Yen, T.L., Hsu W.H. et al. 2013. A novel bioactivity of andrographolide from andrographis paniculata on cerebral ischemia/reperfusion-induced brain injury through induction of cerebral endothelial cell apoptosis. Pharm Biol. 51, 1150–1157.

Wu C, Liu Y, Yang Y, et al. Analysis of therapeutic targets for SARS-CoV-2 and discovery of potential drugs by computational methods. Acta Pharm Sin B. 2020.

Chapter 3 The Virus Slayer

Sukanth KE, Kavitha R et al. Andrographolide as a potential inhibitor of SARS-CoV-2 main protease: an in silico approach. J Biomol Struct Dyn. 2020 : 1–7. Published online 2020 May 5.

Calabrese, C., Berman, S.H. et al. 2000. A Phase 1 Trial of Andrographolide in HIV Positive Patients and Normal Volunteers. Phytotherapy Research 14, 333–338.

Gabrielian, E.S., Panossian, A., et al. 2002. A double blind, placebo controlled study of andrographis paniculata Fixed combination Kan Jang in the treatment of acute upper respiratory tract infections including sinusitis. Phytomedicine 9, 589–597.

Hu, X.Y., Wu, R.H. et al. 2017. Andrographis paniculata (Chuan Xin Lian) for symptomatic relief of acute respiratory infections in adults and children: A systematic review and meta-analysis. PLos 12(8) e0181780.

Naik, S.R., Hule, A. 2009. Evaluation of immunomodulatory activity of an extract of andrographolides from andrographis paniculata. Planta Med. 75, 785–791.

Churiyah X, Pongtuluran O et al. 2015. Antiviral and immunostimulant activities of andrographis paniculata. Journ of Bios 22:2, 67–72.

Saxena, R.C., Singh, R. et al. 2010. A randomized double blind placebo controlled clinical evaluation of extract of andrographis paniculata in patients with uncomplicated upper respiratory tract infection. Phytomedicine 17, 178–85.

Seniya C, Shrivastava S, Singh SK et al 2014, Analyzing the interaction of a herbal compound Andrographolide from andrographis paniculata as a folklore against swine flu (H1N1). Asian Pac J Trop Dis. 2014 Sep;4:S624-S630.

Chapter 4: More Power Against Infections

Calabrese, C., Berman, S.H. et al. 2000. A Phase 1 Trial of Andrographolide in HIV Positive Patients and Normal Volunteers. Phytotherapy Research 14, 333–338.

Chapter 5: Melatonin Gives You More Than ZZZs

Bannerjee, A, Czinn SJ et al. Crosstalk between endoplasmic reticulum stress and anti-viral activities: A novel therapeutic target for COVID-19. Life Sci. 2020 Aug 15; 255: 117842.

Silvestri M, Rossi GA, Melatonin: its possible role in the management of viral infections-a brief review. Ital J Pediatr. 2013; 39: 61.

Srinivasan, V., Maestroni, G., Cardinali, D. et al. Melatonin, immune function and aging. Immun Ageing 2, 17 (2005). https://doi.org/10.1186/1742-4933-2-17

Sanchez-Barcelo, EJ, Mediavilla Md et al. Clinical Uses of Melatonin: Evaluation in Human Trials. Current Medicinal Chemistry, 2020, 17, 2070–2095.

Miller SC, Pandi, PSR et al. The role of melatonin in immuno-enhancement: potential application in cancer. Int J Exp Pathol. 2006 Apr; 87(2): 81–87.

Chapter 6: Ramp Up Your Immune System

Cardoso BR, Apolinario D, Bandeira BS et al. Effects of Brazil nut consumption on selenium status and cognitive performance in older adults with mild cognitive impairment: a randomized controlled pilot trial. European Journal of Nutrition volume 55: 107–116(2016).

Wang MX, Win SS, Pang J. Zinc Supplementation Reduces Common Cold Duration among Healthy Adults: A Systematic Review of Randomized Controlled Trials with Micronutrients Supplementation. Am J Trop Med Hyg. 2020 Apr 27.

Rayman MP. Selenium and Human Health. Lancet. 2012 Mar 31;379(9822): 1256–68.

Chapter 7: Shore Up Liver Function

Chturvedi, G.N., Tomar, G.S. et al. 1983. Clinical studies on Kalmegh (andrographis paniculata nees) in Infective Hepatitis. Anc Sci Life. 2, 208–215.

Mishra, K., Dash, A. et al. 2009. Anti-malarial activities of andrographis paniculata and Hedyotis corymbosa extracts and their combination with curcumin. Malar J. 8: 26.

Sandborn, W.J., Targan, S.R. et al. 2013. Andrographis paniculata extract (HMPL-004) for active ulcerative colitis. Am J Gastroenterol. 108, 90–98.

Toppo, E., Darvin, S. 2016. Effect of two andrographolide derivatives on cellular and rodent models of non-alcoholic fatty liver disease. Molecules. 21:8.

Chapter 8: The Cancer Warrior

Khan, I., Khan, F. et al. 2018. Andrographolide Exhibits Anticancer Potential Against Human Colon Cancer Cells by Inducing Cell Cycle Arrest and Programmed Cell Death via Augmentation of Intracellular Reactive Oxygen Species Level. Nutr Cancer. 70, 787–803.

Seo, E-J., Klauck, S.M., Efferth T., Panossian A. 2019. Adaptogens in chemobrain (Part I): Plant extracts attenuate cancer chemotherapy induced cognitive impairment—Transcriptome-wide microarray profiles of neuroglia cells. Phytomedicine 55, 80–91.

Seo EJ, Klauck SM, Efferth T, Panossian A. Adaptogens in chemobrain (Part II): Effect of plant extracts on chemotherapy-induced cytotoxicity in neuroglia cells. Phytomedicine. 2019b; 58:152743.

Seo, E.J., Klauck, S.M., Efferth, T., Panossian, A. 2019. Adaptogens in chemobrain (Part III): Antitoxic effects of plant extracts towards cancer chemotherapy-induced toxicity—transcriptome-wide microarray analysis of neuroglia cells. Phytomedicine, 56, 246–260.

Chapter 9: The Prince of Hearts

Amroyan, E., Gabrielian, E., Panossian, A., Wikman, G., Wagner, H. 1999. Inhibitory effect of andrographolide from andrographis paniculata on PAF-induced platelet aggregation, Phytomedicine 6, 27–31.

Phunikhom, K., Khampitak, K. 2015. Effect of andrographis paniculata Extract on Triglyceride Levels of the Patients with Hypertriglyceridemia: A Randomized Controlled Trial. J Med Assoc Thai. 98, Suppl 6:S41–7.

Ter-Grigoryan, V., Panossian, A., et al. 2003. Comparative evaluation of the efficacy and safety of multiple doses of Cardiohealth™ in comparison with Renitec™ in patients with mild to moderate hypertension. In: 3rd International Symposium on Natural Drugs. Proceedings, Eds. F.Borelli, F.Capasso, N.Milic, A.Russo. Naples, 2–4 October 2003, Grafidea S.r.l..Milano. pp. 223–226.

Lin KH, Marthandam AS, Kuo WW et a. 2020. Andrographolide mitigates cardiac apoptosis to provide cardio-protection in high-fat-diet-induced obese mice. Environ Toxicol. 2020 Feb 5.

Chapter 10: The Energy Wizard

Rivera. D.S., Lindsay, S. et al. 2016. Andrographolide recovers cognitive impairment in a natural model of Alzheimer's disease (Octodon degus). Neurobiol Aging. 46,204–220.

Thakur, A.K., Rai, G. et al. 2015. Beneficial effects of an andrographis paniculata extract and andrographolide on cognitive functions in streptozotocin-induced diabetic rats. Pharm Biol. 54, 1528–1538.

Dimpfel W, Schombert L, Keplinger-Dimpfelk JK, Panossian A. 2020. Effects of an Adaptogenic Extract on Electrical Activity of the Brain in Elderly Subjects with Mild Cognitive Impairment: A Randomized, Double-Blind, Placebo-Controlled, Two-Armed Cross-Over Study. Pharmaceuticals (Basel). 2020 Mar 14;13(3). pii: E45. doi: 10.3390/ph13030045.

Thakur, A.K., Soni, U.K. et al. 2016. Protective effects of andrographis paniculata extract and pure andrographolide against chronic stress-triggered pathologies in rats. BMC Neurol. 16:77.

Links for Ayurvedic uses

https://www.ncbi.nlm.nih.gov/pmc/articles/PMC4032030/

https://easyayurveda.com/2017/03/08/kalamegha-bhunimba-andrographis-paniculata/

About the Authors

Alexander Panossian Ph.D., Dr.Sc.

Dr. Panossian has multiple advanced degrees in bioorganic chemistry and chemistry of natural and physiologically active compounds. He completed his doctorate in organic chemistry at the Yerevan State University in Armenia in 1971 and obtained his scientific degrees from Moscow Institute of Bioorganic Chemistry in 1975 and Moscow Institute of Fine Chemical Technology in 1986.

His professional positions include the National Academy of Sciences (Armenia, 1975–1986) and the National Institute of Health (Armenia, 1986–1993).

Dr. Panossian was made a full professor of bioorganic chemistry and chemistry of natural and physiologically active compounds in the Russian Federation, and later served as Director of the Laboratory of Quality Control of Drugs of Medical Drug Agency of the Republic of Armenia (1993–2003).

In 2003, he moved to Sweden to act as head of research and development at the Swedish Herbal Institute. He has the honor of participating as a guest scientist in the Laboratory of Nobel Laureate Bengt Samuelsson at the Karolinska Institute in Stockholm (1982–83), at Munich University (1993–95), and at King College in London, 1996. He was the co-editor and the editor-in-chief of Phytomedicine, International Journal of Phytopharmacology and Phytotherapy (Elsevier, Germany) from 2014–2017.

Dr. Panossian is currently Director of Phytomed AB in Sweden. He has authored or co-authored over 180 articles in peer-reviewed journals. His main research interest is focused on plant adaptogens, anti-stress compounds that are involved in the regulation of neuroendocrine and immune system.

Terry Lemerond

Terry Lemerond is a natural health expert with over 50 years of experience helping people live healthier, happier lives. A much sought-after speaker and accomplished author, Terry shares his wealth of experience and knowledge in health and nutrition through his educational programs, including the Terry Talks Nutrition website—TerryTalksNutrition.com—newsletters, podcasts, webinars, and personal speaking engagements. Terry has also hosted Terry Talks Nutrition radio show for the past 30 years. His books include Seven Keys to Vibrant Health, Seven Keys to Unlimited Personal Achievement, and 50+ Natural Health Secrets Proven to Change Your Life. Terry continues to author and co-author books to educate everyone on the steps they can take to live a more vibrant life.

His continual dedication, energy, and zeal are part of his ongoing mission—to help everyone improve their health.

Internet Links

https://www.researchgate.net/profile/Alexander_Panossian2

http://loop.frontiersin.org/people/42293/overview

https://scholar.google.se/citations?user=wJXh8kwAAAAJ&hl=en

https://www.linkedin.com/pub/alexander-panossian/46/a33/555

Index

KNOWLEDGE IS POWER,
ESPECIALLY FOR YOUR HEALTH!

Are you in search of a reliable, science-based resource for all your health and nutrition questions? Terry Talks Nutrition has you covered.

Connect with Terry to increase your knowledge on a wide variety of topics, including immunity, pain, curcumin and cancer, diabetes, and so much more!

READ
Visit TerryTalksNutrition.com for today's latest and greatest health and nutrition information.

LISTEN
Tune in on Sat. and Sun. 8-9 am (CST) at TerryTalksNutrition.com for a live internet radio show hosted by Terry! You can listen to past shows on the website or on your favorite podcast app.

ENGAGE
Connect with us on Facebook, where you can engage with other individuals seeking safe and effective ways to improve overall wellness.

WATCH
Check out our educational YouTube Channel to learn from the world's leading doctors and health experts.

Simply open your smartphone camera. Hold over desired code above for more information.

Get answers to all of your health questions at **TERRYTALKSNUTRITION.COM**

WELCOME TO

ttn
publishing

Are you ready to learn how anyone can use natural medicines, safely and effectively, to improve their health? You'll love TTN Publishing, my newest endeavor to bring you cutting edge research on powerful, health-supporting botanicals. I've coauthored numerous books with top alternative doctors from around the world to help you learn all you can about taking your health into your own hands. These educational books, supported by powerful scientific research, contain all the information you need to live a life of vibrant health.

In Good Health,
Terry Lemerond

BROUGHT TO YOU BY TTN PUBLISHING:

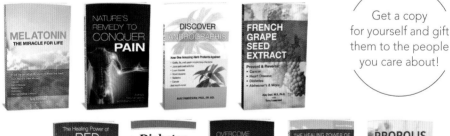

Get a copy for yourself and gift them to the people you care about!

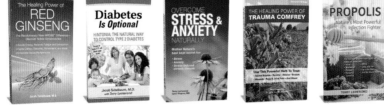

Available at your local health food store or online.

Visit TTNPublishing.com for more news and our latest publications.

TTNPUBLISHING.COM | info@ttnpublishing.com